Bert Hellinger

Pure Consciousness

Paths of Love

Hellinger
PUBLICATIONS

10 9 8 7 6 5 4 3 2 1
2013 2012 2011 2010

Published by
Hellinger
PUBLICATIONS

Sonnleitstr. 37
83404 Bischofswiesen • Germany
Postfach 2120
83462 Berchtesgaden
www.hellinger.com

Cover / Design:
Paper@Screen • Anna W. Moderegger
www.paperscreen.tv

ISBN 978 -3-00-029321-4

Translated by
ANGELIKA SCHENK
Revised and edited by
SUZI TUCKER

Porträt: Riccardo Desiderio
ww.riccardodesiderio.com

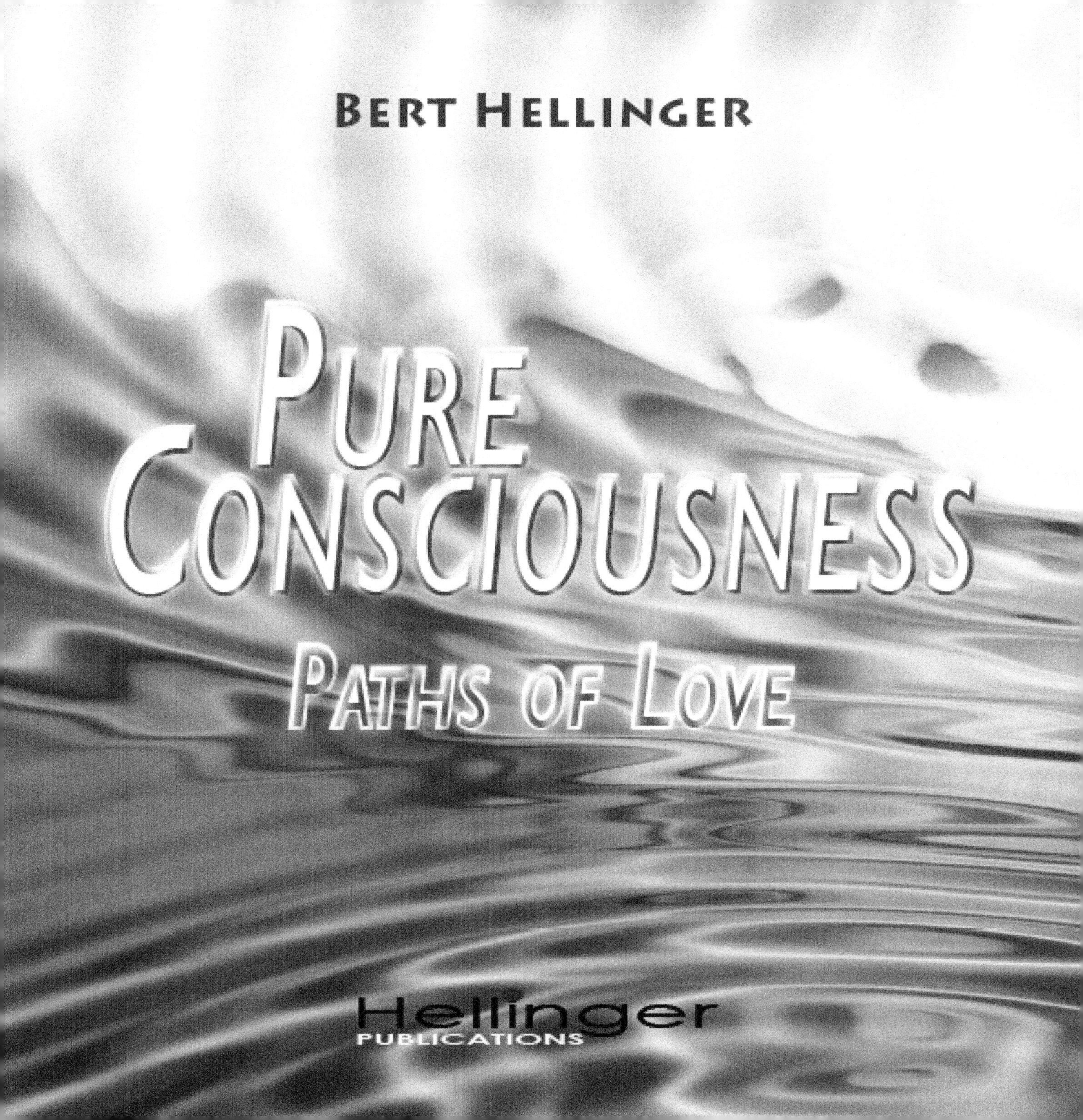

BERT HELLINGER

PURE CONSCIOUSNESS

PATHS OF LOVE

Hellinger
PUBLICATIONS

Inhalt

HOW SHALL I LIFT IT OVER YOU TO OTHER THINGS?

OH HOW I'D LOVE TO HIDE IT IN THE DARK, WITH SOME LOST THING, IN SOME STRANGE SILENT PLACE THAT WILL NOT RESONATE WHEN YOUR DEPTHS ARE SOUNDING FORTH

BUT ANYTHING THAT TOUCHES US, BOTH YOU AND ME, TAKES US TOGETHER IN A SINGLE BOWING THAT DRAWS FROM TWO STRINGS BUT ONE VOICE.

ON WHOSE INSTRUMENT ARE WE STRUNG? AND WHICH FIDDLER HOLDS US IN HIS HAND?

O SWEET SONG

GUIDE TO BERT HELLINGER'S PUBLICATIONS IN ENGLISH

Introduction
Pure consciousness

Pure consciousness is directed towards actions in the service of love and life, in a way that everything opposing them is left behind.

Pure consciousness remains beyond anything that could cloud it. It remains outside of personal intentions that would allow one's own interests to oppose the spiritual movement that is working in every life and in love, and taking them to their fulfillment in the end.

The chapters in this book are concerned with this way of taking action. They describe what serves it, and they take you along into this way of acting, beginning with first steps, until pure consciousness guides you on your pure path, taking your life to a pure goal, together with your love.

All contemplations in this book come from personal experience and lead to personal experience for those taken along on this path, gladly so, in their own personal way. This purity is an experience of fullness, it comes at the end of a path. On this path it will accompany us further and further. Hence, all that's required is taking the first few steps.

In this book, I'll join you for a while until you continue your journey on your own, to where your purity is taking you, into your pure love, your fulfilled life, and your pure happiness.

Bert Hellinger

HOW SHALL
I HOLD
MY SOUL
SO THAT IT IS NOT
TOUCHING YOURS?

Conscious

Conscious means, I know something in a way that it guides me, I know what needs to be done and what consequences it will have.

Because I am aware of it, I own up to it, without making excuses or deviating from it.

When I become aware of something I did not know before, it comes as a surprise. For now I see a connection that allows me to respond and act in new ways. Now I might be able to restore something into order, a relationship for instance. In this sense my consciousness expands. It becomes wider and deeper, it includes more.

When something remains unclear, we sometimes speak of a clouded perception. Especially when we prefer not to acknowledge something. So the expansion of consciousness has something to do with our willingness to face reality as it is, no matter how painful and challenging it may be.

This growth of consciousness is preceded by a purification. This means a farewell to expectations that exceed what is possible, and a farewell to images of reality that are in contradiction to clear thinking.

Above all this consciousness presupposes that we agree to reality as it is, that we are also willing to submit to it. In consenting to it, we understand it more deeply and more purely.

In consenting, we also become more aware of our limitations. Accepting our limits and remaining within the scope of our possibilities, we become naturally modest.

Above all, this consciousness is pure. It comes with love.

Pure and simple

On the one hand, what's simple is easy, easy to understand and easy to deal with. On the other hand simplicity is the nature of essential things, everything essential is simple.

Everything important in life is simple. It serves life through its very simplicity.

The essential word is clear and easy to take in. It limits itself to what works immediately. Great thoughts are simple, and so is great love. Anything it wants, anywhere it leads, is clear and straightforward. The pure and simple expects little and offers much.

Taste is sometimes plain and simple, and in this sense what is simple is also unassuming, unpretentious. Simplicity supports immediate connection with others because it does not stand out from others. It is barely noticed.

A yes or a no, accepting an offer or declining it, such statements are clear and binding. In the past, a simple handshake often sufficed to express a clear commitment.

Only the pure and simple has fullness, the fullness of life, for what's pure and simple is in accord with many things. Being simple, straightforward and to the point, it forms connections easily.

As such, the simple life is the full life. It does not waste importance on trivialities, and hence it remains free for what matters.

Pure consciousness

Pure consciousness is complete consciousness. It contains everything at once. This consciousness is all- embracing because it includes everything without preferences and gives equal attention to everything. Any distinctions in the sense of preferences of one over the other would cloud it.

In pure consciousness everything is connected with everything else within a system of order. This means, in pure consciousness everything has its proper place, its own place, together with many other things that also have their proper place.

For pure consciousness everything is equally in existence. Everything is there in its right place, and therefore everything is in order as it is.

Pure consciousness is pure because it does not exclude anything from its kind attention. It is directed towards everything at the same time, equally awake and clear in its presence for everything.

Because pure consciousness encompasses everything, it remains without images, for images would limit it. Where is does form and work through images, these images are there for all equally; they are open images, wide images, images that remain general and therefore speak to all.

The same spirit is at work when pure consciousness expresses itself. It finds the right words, words that go to the heart of the matter, words that create something new.

Pure consciousness remains in motion, in a pure movement; pure, for the creatively new is only just coming. It comes immediately out of this consciousness, without any prior connection to anything. Accordingly, the new arising out of this consciousness is also pure, pure in the sense of immediate, and pure also as an existence of its own, whole in itself.

Which consciousness did I speak of here? Can it be my consciousness? As I could speak about it, I was connected to it, connected thus that it reveals itself as a pure consciousness in me as well, and that I experience myself as pure through this consciousness.

Though we come from this consciousness, it is also our journey's destination. We are on the way in purity, for we are drawn into this pure consciousness, taken along by it. Step by step we experience greater purity because we are also including more and more in our attention, taking it along in increasing purity, purely as it is.

In this consciousness our love becomes pure, too. It becomes pure because we remain in our own place within the whole in purity; pure, as we remain within the order of this pure consciousness; pure, as our love also brings about new things in its creativity; pure, as our love is there in its purity, fully there, equally and steadily there; awake, and yet, calmly resting in this other consciousness.

Evening

"Evening's stillness everywhere", is the beginning of a song. In the evening the day finds rest. It gets tired and falls asleep.

Evening is the time of looking back. We feel calm now when the day brought and achieved something so that we look back at it feeling fulfilled, grateful for what it brought and gave us.

In the evening we let go. Taking our time to let the day fade away, we begin to prepare ourselves for the night.

What happens after the evening, in the night? The night takes us into another realm, away from the day. The evening was only the transition into the night.

What was only transitory, and too much for the day, begins only in the night. The day really only ends in the night. For not the day, but the night takes us further.

In the evening we move between these two realms. The day flows over into the night and ends in it. When we wake up again, it's a new day, a different day.

The evening already gives us a dim sense of the new day, but first the night pushes in between the two days.

Where is our home? Is it the day or the night?

In the evening we find ourselves in between the two. It is neither day nor night. It is transition time, until sleep overcomes us. Only our sleep closes the day off. Only then does the new begin. It begins in our sleep. Only with the beginning of the new is the day completely over.

The abyss

The abyss that scares us the most is the one inside of us. We recoil from it. We are afraid of falling into it and being devoured by it.

We fight against the vortex that might pull us into the abyss. We also try to deny this pull, pretending it did not exist for us. We refuse to admit to it, through countermeasures, like good deeds and friendliness, through visible and tangible love.

Yet behind them the eeriness of our abyss is lying in wait. For fear of it we change the way we live, sometimes we carry on as if it did not exist. But obviously the good in us is still fed and spurred on through our defense against the pull and the might of our inner abyss.

What is the effect our abyss has on us in the long run? Without our inner abyss, would we have what it takes to serve life and further it? Why would we beseech God's love without the simultaneous fear of His abyss? Of hell, for example? Can we think of a deeper abyss?

But why does hell fascinate us in so many inner and outer images? Is hell God's abyss? Is it ours? Is the fear of God our fear?

Nevertheless, our abyss is a blessing. It cautions us and protects us from the fall we fear. It walks with us wherever we love, wherever we serve. It keeps us wake.

The more we try to rise above it, the more it draws us close to it and downwards. From the abyss we gain the power that builds on it, fearing as well as acknowledging and loving it.

Grateful

Being grateful means, I acknowledge and take what I was given, exactly as I have it. It fulfills me as it is.

What happens in the moment of such gratefulness? I release those who gave so much to me from any further expectations. For instance my mother and father.

Where I want more, my gratitude becomes empty. Only when my gratitude means that I feel fulfilled through what I received, that I now take what I already have, only then does it make me rich for my future.

The same holds true for other relationships, like with our partner. When I gratefully release my partner from special expectations, I set him or her free to remain in close connection with me.

Relating with gratitude means, becoming free through receiving, setting free through receiving.

Gratitude means, receiving and taking it with love, in order to pass on with love. Gratitude frees us for further loving relationships. Where we succeeded in grateful receiving from our parents, we are free to give in other relationships.

Our relationships begin with mutual giving and taking. Later on a time comes where this relationship is fulfilled in many regards, so that we can say to our partner something like what we said to our mother and father: "Thank you, you have given me such riches, so much that I set you free from the depth of my soul."

From then on both are on a different level, separated as well as one. They are separated with gratitude and yet one in love in a new way. The inner expectations we used to have ceased to be. All the more our further giving and taking remains free and open for new ways.

This love is transmuted. It is one with something greater. It is like devotion, recollected and still, like our love before God.

Service

Service furthers something. In service we help others to live their life in a better way. Our service supports their life. Through my service others can grow and live better, more carefree and lighter.

The question is, when we serve others, does it really serve them? Does it make them fitter to deal with life in good ways? Or is our serving others similar to the way a mother looks after her child, even when this child already has the strength to live independently, capable of succeeding out of its own strength, achieving what serves life? Does our helping hinder others in their growth because we want to support their growth more than our own? Do we serve others from the mindset of a child that finds it hard to bear their parents' suffering? Do we overlook that each one of us has the key to their own treasure box, that no one else can open it?

Serving means, remaining in accord with a movement of life in which we are constantly engaged in helping one another, mutually supporting our life. In harmony with these movements we also leave others the space needed for their own unfoldment, the personal space that must be expanded and deepened through their own strength, in order to live life fully. Only then can we support the lives of others in shared living.

So how do we conduct ourselves, when others serve us? We accept their serving, often unquestioned, like children taking from their parents. At the same time we set a limit to their serving, where any further help would mean a limit to the unfoldment of their and our lives. This limit we all have to overcome ourselves.

Serving is ultimately living life, living our own life and serving the life that is to come, until this coming life in its turn serves future life as well.

Equanimity

Equanimity is a noble state of mind, because it remains kindly turned to everyone on the same level, with goodwill towards them and itself. Therefore, what comes from others, is also received with equanimity. It will not get drawn into anything, for everything must be the received equally by the mind poised in the centre. Everything is left with those to whom it belongs, with goodwill and yet in all clarity.

The equanimous ones give everything equal importance, knowing everything as basically transient, already seeing the time when a given thing is less important. This means, they let it go now so that they remain free from it, even if they engage in the matter right now. They leave things their importance just for now, equanimously.

Those of equal mind know whatever comes will also pass in its due time. So they serve everything in passing, within the appointed boundaries. They remain equanimous, coming and going themselves, like everything else.

Great love is equanimous, too. It is there any time, while it lasts. It may also depart when its time has come. But it gazes after the other with unchanged love, with equal minded love, for it remains as it was.

For the equanimous ones everything is coming as well as going, and so are they, coming and going in their own time, there and not there, on the road with everything and everyone that is coming and going as they do.

Spirit, above all, is of equal mind. For spirit everything has its own time, yet nothing is ever lost. Spirit's love is unwavering in all things, kindly turned to everything, with unwavering love, without preferences. Everyone and everything is equally loved, equally accepted, equally received, equally arriving at the one destination.

The jester

The fool has a certain degree of freedom. In one way he is important. He expresses what others are not allowed to say. At the same time, dressed up as a fool, he it only taken seriously in a superficial way. Serious matters he expresses are presented in fool's robes.

Sometimes we also express something we really mean, just as a passing remark, nearly like a joke. This way we masquerade as a fool, and so remain protected from many attacks. "He's a clown", say those in self protection who could otherwise feel targeted by the fool's words. It appears to be a game, a light-hearted game, even though it is serious.

Sometimes the fool was also ordered to be the taster. He had to taste his master's food to check if it safe.

A poisoned fool seemed like a small misfortune since the master's life was saved.

Here it shows, before the fool had to swallow the poison, he had to swallow the truth and test it out on himself. He knew his days were numbered anyhow. Is that the reason he was so funny?

On the other hand the fool's performance demonstrated that a naked truth could be concealed under the fool's garment. Everything else was a game – a gamble with his life at stake, though.

What reveals itself in the fool and under his garment? A dreaded truth, still made a fool of by many and yet already revealed in its concealed form.

What do many festive garments and robes turn out to be? A mere appearance that has a truth hidden behind it, dressed up as something else, for a time, until its robes fall, too.

Fog

The fog takes our vision away. Often it sits on the land in a thick, heavy layer, especially in the low lying areas, and over rivers and lakes. Only higher up does the fog begin to clear, and there we can see clearly again.

We also talk about fog, when something remains impenetrable for us. We can't see what's going on any more. Sometimes certain things are also being clouded deliberately, to prevent people from seeing clearly what is going on; in a war for instance.

When we want to hide something from others, we express ourselves vaguely, unclearly, so that they can't understand what we are on about. What we say remains foggy for them; rather than telling them something, we cover it up, and they are easily lead on a wrong track.

How do we deal with such a situation? We wait for the fog to clear, or perhaps also for the other side to lose their orientation in their fog, so that we might even look for a way out together. Or when we feel thoroughly disorientated in thick fog, we go higher up. Here we gain an overview and find our direction and our path again- sometimes also for others.

What above all, clouds our spirit? Many wishes, demands, and expectations of others, and the offers of those who make out they could fulfill them. In this way, many a hope ends up in fog.

In contrast to this, the present moment is clearly before us, and what it has to offer. Clear is the love that stays with what is nearby, clear is the joy and the happiness now. Happiness shines bright and clear as the sun.

Whatever furthers life is clear, and clear is the live that serves it. Clear is the decisive insight, that reveals many things in a new light.

Clear is elucidation and enlightening education which places the absurd into the light of reason, thereby stripping it of its power.

Clear is our consenting to everything that is and how it is. Nothing eschews it. Clear above all is the eternal, the eternal now.

Development

Everything alive develops from small beginnings to full maturity. A tree starts out as a seed. The seed already contains the blueprint of its development. All it has to do is unfold.

It is the same for human beings. The fertilized egg already contains its development. The whole human being is its unfoldment.

This development is already given for every living being. Only unfolding in this preordained way, will it be able to pass life on. So this unfolding goes way beyond the individual life. It is embedded in a large field of development and evolution, in the development of its species and kind, for instance.

Thus humanity develops as a whole, on many levels. Together with humanity, the world in which we live develops also. The development of individual living beings is embedded in this all encompassing development, in which everything and everyone is dependent on each other, all contributing to this development.

An aspect of this development is, that the individual living beings all make room for those who come after them. For the individual, including the human individual, only makes a limited contribution to this overall development, especially in passing its life on to the next generation. Therefore the individual also undergoes a kind of devolution. When its work is done its strength fades, it lessens and weakens, withers and dies. Seen from the whole this is also a part of evolution. Individual evolution comes to a limit that the individual cannot go beyond. The individual's development can only continue on in its descendents. They take the next steps.

But within a life span we experience personal growth. Again, not in isolation, but together with many others, with humanity and the world as a whole. We develop in accord with the whole and in mutual giving and taking. In this way our personal development becomes a service to the whole. Development therefore means serving. Every development moves towards serving. It reaches fulfillment in serving, as it is orientated to serving something greater.

How do we look at ourselves then? How do we look at others? How do we look at the world and all of creation?

We see the whole in evolution. We see all beings and all things, all of creation embedded in an evolution, and we agree to this evolution.

In this perspective we see ourselves and everything else differently, we relate differently to ourselves and to others, and to the world we live in.

Whatever there is and was, that we bumped against, as it is and as it was, is was and is a part of something that was and is in service of some development. Therefore it is not our place to want things differently in the past or the present. We do not know what it needs to contribute to. Consenting to whatever is developed further this way, wherever it leads, we grow as well. We remain in accord with the powers at work behind every development, willing things as they are, as they come about, our development, the development of those close to us, and any development wherever it leads us, together with all else.

Agreeing thus, we set ourselves and others free from everything that runs counter to this accord. This agreeing to everything as it is, as it develops, is love, love for everything as it moves on and as it serves the development of everything and everyone.

Bringing together

What can be joined in, fits in. Fitting in well, it stays in place well, like for instance the keystone in a vault.

This is an external image of a good fit. It closes a gap.

In our life, too, many things fit in well; many gaps are closed. It is the same here, when things come together that fit well. Something comes together well in a partner relationship. Marriage for a couple is like placing the keystone, turning two half arches into a whole one that will be strong and stable from hereon.

In a jigsaw puzzle, the last piece completes the whole picture. Therefore we search carefully for the place where it will fit in exactly. This is also an image for processes in science. Many people do research for a certain project and find many different building blocks. But only when the last brick has been found that joins everything into a whole, stability is achieved, and the can researchers complete their work on something so that it lasts, to be built upon and used. Here again, the last missing link is essential. When everything fits in, the resulting whole is durable, and it can be applied successfully.

Here, the joining together is the result of an achievement that took many people a lot of effort.

Many things come together like this in our life, in surprising, often unforeseeable ways. We experience it as a gift, provided from elsewhere.

For instance, a decisive insight is such a gift of providence. When we come into accord with the powers that guide and lead us every step on the way, we expect happy coincidences every day.

Sometimes we are waiting for such a coincidence sent from above. But it comes in its own time, at the right time. It is testing our trust.

As a rule, providence delivers the missing link differently to what we expected, for it is in the service of powers that have other things in mind than what we superficially wish for. In the end, this bringing together shows itself as love for many. We experience this gift as peace. Finally the conflict is over, all breathe a deep sigh of relief. In the service of this movement we also succeed in bringing things together for the good of many. How? With love.

Interfering

What do people usually interfere with? With something that is not their business. They interfere even though they have not earned the right to be involved. Nor are they ready to take responsibility for their interference.

This is how many people meddle in the lives of others, even in their intimate feelings and innermost thoughts; sometimes also with their health. Like giving advice the consequences of which have to be born by the other person, not by the meddlers.

In this meddling, where is the respect for the other person, where is the love? Is there any understanding and acceptance of our limits? Where is the respect for the insight and the achievement that is there for the other person to gain?

Many objections belong to this kind of meddling. They want to impede or limit something, often without knowing the issue.

The opposite to meddling is support. Support furthers a movement, it contributes to a good outcome and is happy about a success. Different to meddling, support brings things together, instead of causing separation. Meddlers end up being on their own.

But there is also a beneficial intervention. In case of fire we are glad to see the fire brigade arrive. In contrast to interfering through objections which is usually cheap, interfering with a fire is costly. It asks the ultimate of those engaged in the operation, sometimes even their lives.

A helpful interference is the law that sets boundaries to a range of interferences. Giving people important information, providing insightful education, these are also useful interventions. For instance, they free us from religions that want to interfere with our relationship to God, like when they claim to have the right of dictating to us what takes us closer to God and what takes us away from Him.

It is similar in regards to the public moral code. How many people meddle with the lives of others in the name of morals, especially in the lives of children!

How do we remain in love? When we renounce meddling. All of a sudden other forces are set free, original, beneficial, inspiring, creative forces – in us and in others.

Upwards

The priests and the congregation sing in holy mass: "Raise up your hearts. We have them with the Lord." This song describes a basic movement that lifts us beyond ourselves into another realm. Here a creative power can be experienced that carries us beyond our life, towards a destination. Deep down we know we are already on the way, we sense that this power is taking us along even now.

"Raise up your hearts" is a movement of joy. It removes our earthly heaviness and sets something in motion inside us, and we have a sense of lightness. It lifts us above many things in our daily life, into a movement beyond, where we are connected with many others in love.

This movement is a movement of the spirit and a movement of the heart. It's a pulsating movement, full of power. Compared to this experience, everything that pulls us down is old and weak.

Together with the spirit, our thoughts are raised, too, they become lofty thoughts, sublime thoughts, wide open thoughts. They lift us beyond the realm of heaviness, into the consciousness that encompasses all, into a pure consciousness, free from all kinds of burdens.

Our body is also directed upwards. Walking upright has the same effect on us as the spirit. It also draws our body away from gravity's downward pull, and into an upward movement, beyond earth's heaviness. Our body is also taken along into this upward movement, into a movement of getting up, standing tall, and rising from the dead, upwards to spirit.

Up above we are at home, up there we will stay, there where our heart has been all along.

This upward movement is a movement of love. A love for whom? The love for all, the love that this spirit draws towards itself. How? Upwards.

Relieved

Sometimes we take on something that burdens us, and after some time we realize that it is too heavy for us or out of place. Then we secretly hope for something to magically happen that will relieve us from this burden. We take a deep breath when we can return to what is in accord with our own life. We got rid of something and we became free for something else, for something of our own.

We also feel relieved when we got rid of a sense of guilt or of an obligation that does not belong to us, something that someone else incurred, yet we had to take it on and bear the consequences.

The same applies in reverse. We also remain within our boundaries in our connections with others and respect theirs. This means we carry the consequences of our behavior ourselves instead of burdening others with them. Where we have burdened others, we relieve them of it, by releasing them from our expectations and demands.

Having learnt form our experiences, how do we safeguard our boundaries and our independence for the future? Neither do we interfere in the domains of others nor do we allow others to interfere in ours.

Does this separate us from others? Does it separate others from us? In a certain way it does, but in a wholesome way. From here on, we meet others as equals, connected and still free. Free for joint endeavors where everyone gives and takes, but in accord with a common goal, a shared task, a shared obligation, in accord with mutual respect and love, in accord with a love that is free to love.

Following

Following can mean two things. One, there is a law, or I receive an order. So I follow by obeying it, I behave in accord with it. This way I give up something of myself. I submit to an external order that I am delivered to.

Following also means, I follow in the footsteps of someone who walks ahead of me. This can be meant literally, when I obediently follow a leader who guides me on a path yet unfamiliar to me. I happily follow because this path is important to me. This leader walks in front of me. He shows me the path he knows and walks himself. In a certain way he serves me. He helps me on.

I also follow a personal impulse, a personal desire, a personal wish. Here I follow something I want or need. Often this can be essential for my life. To quite an extent, it is dictated to me, so I obediently follow, out of personal need. Like this we also pursue an instinctual urge.

When it comes to wishes we often have a choice whether to pursue them or not. Therefore we check to what extent a wish can be fulfilled, and at what price. Only then do we decide if we want to pursue this wish and pay the ensuing price for it.

We also follow a sudden insight and a personal destiny. We do it with a sense of being guided. This guidance comes from a spiritual power that grabs hold of our innermost self and takes us along with it. Being allowed to follow it, feels like a gift. Through this gift we are taken along into a direction that bestows meaning on our life, beyond its daily pursuits and needs. We follow it, in accord with it, against all superficial objections. In this following, we experience ourselves fulfilled.

HOW SHALL
I LIFT IT OVER YOU
TO OTHER THINGS ?

Heard

When someone calls us, we usually answer: "I hear you." A mother reprimands an unruly child by saying: "Didn't you hear me?" In former times it was considered a principle of education to say to children: "That's what you get for not listening."

Of some people, it was said that they heard the voice of God; Abraham for instance, when God told him to sacrifice his son as a burnt offering. Something similar was said of the prophets and of Jesus. They also said, they had heard the voice of God, and were now proclaiming what they heard from God as God's Words.

Sometimes we also perceive a sudden idea like an inner voice that we heed and act upon.

Such intuitions are sometimes clear and irresistible. We have to follow them. Mothers for instance have such inner impulses. Through their close connections with their children they sometimes know immediately what their child needs. The child might even be somewhere else, yet they still hear its voice when it is in trouble and needs their help.

Such inner messages serve life and love. When we heed them they usually prove to be correct and precise. They are always helpful.

Then there are other inner messages whose origin we can't work out. For instance when someone feels called upon to start a war, often in the name of some higher power or an idea, sweeping many others with them, into perdition. Such inner calls also seem to be irresistible.

How do we deal with such callings when we are swept along, too?

We wait for a personal message from inside. We open our inner ears wide and hearken into the distance. Suddenly we hear what is expected of us. When we follow this personal voice, this personal instruction, we remain composed and calm, and we remain kindly disposed others. What we set out to do as the consequence of this inner contact, will succeed. We succeed in a way helpful to us and others.

After some time we are open to this guidance from inside every step of the way. We live hearing, we answer listening, awake, humble, composed, serving, carried by another consciousness in all matters, always carried in its love with love.

Competent

Competence stands for know-how and skilful application. Competence means both, the knowledge and the practical skills to carry out a task, to solve a problem.

This level of competence is an achievement. It was gained through long periods of learning and practicing. Therefore a competent service comes at a price. Even though expensive at times, it often turns out to be the best deal, offering the best solution.

A person becomes competent through dedicated effort and through a special talent. Most people can't be competent in every regard. Competence in some field requires having an eye for the task, the right flair, knowledge and intuition, and the corresponding physical constitution, skills, dexterity.

Competent people exist in all domains of human activity, gardeners as they deal with plants, a farmer or breeder dealing with livestock, specialists in trades, let alone housewives that run a household, take care of their children, and provide good meals.

People in professional service are often also very competent. For instance good doctors, with an especially extensive range of knowledge and specific skills, or good teachers, organizers, entrepreneurs, salespeople and helpers in various fields.

Great competence is required in the professions of the fine arts, as for instance with architects, painters, sculptors, poets, writers, musicians, film directors. Prerequisites here are highly developed gifts and talents, and a willingness to work hard, practicing for a long time in order to attain mastery in their field.

In any case, ability is far more than just knowledge. It is skillfully applied knowledge that serves many, making their lives easier, richer and more beautiful.

Our greatest and most important skill is the art of living. The essential knowledge and ability we received already at birth. The fundamental needs of life are governed by common needs, instincts, and drives. They help us survive, survive skillfully.

But this alone isn't an art yet. For the art of living it takes lifelong learning and acting, - and it takes love of life, the joy of living life as it is and as it can be sustained and developed further.

Every other competence, every other skill, great or small, serves this art.

Denying

In denying or lying, a person denies or repudiates something. This often happens when others want to coax this person into an admission of something, so that they feel justified in reprimanding or calling to account the person that they corner. Children often lie out of fear of punishment.

Who is really denying something here? Who wants to avoid a truth, who does not want to acknowledge it? Are the questioners in accord with love, with their own and that of others? Does the other person perhaps lie out of a need for self defense, as if their life was at stake? Is this what the lie is all about?

What kind of attitude and behavior would make lying and covering up unnecessary in this situation?

Firstly, the respect for the other person's secret, for their truth.

Secondly, looking at our own truth, so we understand that we also have some secrets to guard, just as others have theirs.

Thirdly, remaining in the love that consents to everything as it is, including our own fear and our own distress. This love also consents to a future that allows us and others, to overcome this distress.

Suddenly we can show ourselves as we are, and the others can do the same. In this trust that comes out of love, we can allow another a glance into our deep secrets, and may be they will reciprocate.

Yet even here, we are still protecting our deepest secrets from unfamiliar glances. We protect them with love.

Separated

Separated means, everyone walks their own path. Our own path is the right path. Only on our own path do we arrive at our destination, in accord with the powers that gave us this path, individually preordained.

Nobody has the right to dictate other people which path to take. When two people walk side by side for some time, as if they had a common path, after a while it becomes apparent that their paths begin to diverge. Then they might try to pull the other person over to their path. They might mutually expect that the other one leave his or her own path and follow that of the partner. Then they both loose a leg of their own path. Even though they still walk together for another stretch of the path, they experience the inner separation from the other.

How do we find our way back to our togetherness and to the love that once was? Strangely as it sounds, we find each other again in separation, for our own individual path connects us most deeply. How? Both follow the same inner voice.

Our separated ways only appear to separate us. In reality we are united in the obedience to the same spiritual power that bids us walk different paths, guided by the spiritual love that wants us individually different. We arrive at agreeing to our separate ways, and become most mindfully united one with another, in the depth of out heart.

Complicated

Something appears complicated to us when we can't find a clear line. Different lines tend to go in different directions, so it's hard for us to gain an overview and to arrive at a shared sense of direction.

In this manner there are complicated marriages, complicated problems, complicated issues, complicated tasks. Where different things have to be bundled for some joint venture and directed to a shared goal, it easily gets complicated for us.

When different spiritual persuasions want to agree to a common direction, it usually does not take very long before it gets too complicated for them to persevere with their enthusiasm.

We observe this for instance with the ecumenical movements within Christian creeds, let alone with occasional attempts of persuading members of different religions to join in some shared project, at least for a preliminary dialogue.

It is easier to maintain some degree of dialogue through making allowances for the difficulties. Then the movements which are still in opposition can agree to each walk their own paths as independent movements with different directions, mutually acknowledging each other without searching or aiming for a common approach in central issues.

In relationships of this kind it gets especially complicated when one partner wants to have the upper hand and get their own way. Mutual tolerance often achieves more in terms of good relationships than an agreement in some abstract middle ground where both sides feel restricted by or delivered to the other side.

The redeeming key sentence is here: The same right and the same freedom of movement for all.

Dear God

"Dear God!" we sigh sometimes, when we are puzzled or distressed about something that happened to us. Hidden in this is a call for help: "God, how could you allow this to happen!" It is also a reproach.

Why do we want God to be good to us, good in the way we want it? Do we want Him to be good especially to us, not so much to others? Do we even want Him to be against others, to oppose them?

How can this God be a dear God when He is only good to some and less so to others, or not at all good to them?

This dear God in this sense is my God, above all, my God. Then I dictate to Him what He has to do, so that He stays my dear God.

It says in the bible: God is Love. What does the bible want to say with this, what does it mean for us? Do we acknowledge, does the bible acknowledge in this statement that God is equally good to all? That in His love He has the same goodwill towards all, no allowing preferences among them? Or do we expect our God to prefer us and even to have ill will against certain others? For instance, by damning them?

How would it be if we asked Him: "Be their dear God, too, be good to them, too."? Is He still our dear God then? Do we still love Him as our God? Or do we feel abandoned by Him, because His love is different to what the child in us would like it to be?

When we submit to Him, the way He loves all equally, us like everyone else, together with them, do we still dare to say: "Dear God"? Or do we, in our innermost self, begin to resonate with His one and the same love for all?

Then our dear God is the God of love for all, including those whom we refused to love until now. Then we submit to His greater love and begin to love as He does. How?

We wish everyone the love of God, as He loves us all, when we begin to love like He does, – loving all equally and all at the same time.

Bait

Bait lures us into a trap. It promises something but it is an empty promise, for it only wants to trap us.

Such bait we find in advertising. The promises made are not always empty- but expensive. They entice us to buy something we do not really need, or that may even be harmful to us, like some medication. Often we realize that we are baited, but we still fall for it.

The most dangerous bait are promises of salvation, combined with the threat that we lose body and life and soul if we do not comply with the conditions that are the imposed requirements for salvation.

Who makes such promises of salvation? People who want to gain power over our soul and spirit: for their own advantage and at our misfortune. Many of these soul ensnarers however, are themselves already the victims of such soul catchers.

How do we eschew the fascinations of such promises of salvation? We observe how they operate:

Firstly, nearly all these promises are postponed into a dim future, so that for this life here they appear hollow and empty.

Secondly, they are tied to conditions that prove to be life restricting, and even life constricting, sometimes deadly so.

Thirdly, these conditions are ascribed to a god who only loves those who fulfill these conditions. Those who don't are excluded from this god's love, and even damned for eternity.

But how can the Creator of all life be wanting something that opposes life, the life that he created? Is not life itself the greatest promise of blessing? Do these ensnarers not catch us against this blessing?

How do we protect ourselves against them? We close our ears to their beckoning call and our eyes in the face of their treacherous glamour. We let life charm us, life as it is, given to us as the greatest revelation. We rejoice in it now as it brings fulfillment every moment. We take it in with love, even now, right now.

Right

In our context here, right means, it is helpful. Whether something is right, is assessed by the result it brings. This has nothing to do with the distinction of right and wrong as defined by criteria and directions we are expected to adhere to, because they serve our belonging to our groups, and therefore our good conscience. Here we speak of right as a measure of helpfulness.

Right in this sense is everything that serves life; everything that helps a human relationship to work well or to work again.

Ultimately, everything that serves love is right. The right move, the right love, they ignore many boundaries of a moral or religious nature. They are oriented towards what allows life – and our happiness – to flourish.

Right has something to do with direction. The right points into a direction that is goal oriented and succeeds in something.

Right in this sense are thoughts pertaining to the matter at hand, in accord with it and supporting its success.

Right is everything that is perceived as real, especially the movement in which something goes and must go.

At this stage the right is often not revealed as yet. This holds true for any creative movement and for the insight it sets in motion. So what is right reveals itself in its movements and in its effects.

What is always right, is the love that creatively effects something new, especially new life. What serves life is therefore always right. This direction reaches the essential goal, even with the goal posts perpetually moving

Inconspicuous

The little flower in the wall is inconspicuous. It has but little room to unfold, and yet it manages to turn itself into something attractive and beautiful. It makes full use of the small space. The small crack in the wall is also fulfilled through something inconspicuous. All the more amazed, we pause to look at it. It draws us to it.

Even in the glamorous we are sometimes looking for some small detail. We may notice something minor that is complete in itself. For the copious and grand becomes tiresome after a while. Then we prefer to take a rest with the rather inconspicuous.

We feel the same about our own inconspicuous. It needs little attention, and it proves itself to be what we are comfortable with in the long run. The inconspicuous clothes we wear at home, for instance.

The inconspicuous leave us and others in peace. It's not in the limelight to be compared to others or commented on. Nobody needs to put it down. Where to? It's down already. It doesn't invite any fuss.

Above all else, spirit is inconspicuous. Who can take hold of it? Who can shine with it? And yet it is present, inconspicuously, as it permeates everything from inside, from a mysterious depth. In accord with its movement, we are present in the same way, remaining inconspicuous, composed, at ease. We remain alert, present, awake to its movement.

Growth is also inconspicuous. Not noticing anything for some time, we suddenly find ourselves amazed about its result, the result of a movement of the spirit. Inconspicuously at work in the background, it is barely noticed, but powerful.

The day to day life of love also lives off the inconspicuous, of the little gestures, the little kindnesses. Nothing is done as an exhibition. Love lives through its existence, it's modest being- there.

In this sense everything of depth is inconspicuous. Deep love, deep devotion, deep trust. Above all, we are inconspicuous before God.

Into the wide open

A path is long when its destination lies in the far distance. Yet the next step is always nearby.

A consciousness is wide when it is open for anything as it shows itself. Our consciousness becomes narrow when it excludes things and restricts its attention to few things.

Wide in this sense is the love that agrees to everything as it is. Wide also means open, open for everything as it shows itself, open for what it takes us to, open also in not knowing where the journey will take us.

Wide open is everything new, because it is still just at the beginning. It remains wide when it moves towards the next new phase. Its movement goes forward as well as into the wide open.

Wide is everything that is permitted to expand, in all directions and dimensions.

Sometimes things reach their destined limitation. A tree for instance can only reach a certain height, but never the sky.

Wide is the gaze when it takes in many things at once. The wide gaze also comes to its limits at the horizon. Still, it goes beyond this boundary to the extent of its eyes' perceptive capacity. For with the help of instruments our gaze moves beyond many boundaries, into the wide open, the higher up, and down to a depth hitherto restricted.

Wide, above all, are our thoughts. Nothing can hinder them, nothing can constrict them. In this regard they are free.

The question is: Is there a corresponding reality? Then this reality becomes a boundary that the thoughts have to submit to.

It is different with the thoughts that become real because they are creative. They effect something that did not exist until then. They go beyond the present boundaries of our possibilities, into a new open space.

What is brought to effect by these thoughts, comes from the far away into the near, when we realize them by taking action. Only in our actions does this far and wide come near, near now, continuously approaching, always in motion. Where to? Into the wide open.

Kind attention

Kindly turned means, I turn to others and I go towards them, with attentive love. Kindly turned to others also means, I turn to people as they are. I let go of my ideas that they should be different to how they are, that their actions and intentions should be different to what is possible for them.

This presupposes that I am also kindly turned to myself, as I am and was. That I also turn kindly to myself with my so called faults and weaknesses, including everything I have burdened others with, every injury and harm I caused them.

How do we succeed in this kind attention? We realize that in every regard each one of us is taken into service by other forces, each one of us in our own way. We come to see the same power at work in everyone. Therefore we understand that it is not our place to consider what is right or wrong for any individual, including ourselves, no matter how people are, how people behave and act, whatever we become aware of in people, including ourselves, now or later. Therefore in our kind attention to others we refrain form anything that might diminish or oppose our kindness through our thoughts and wishes of good or bad.

Something else allows us this kind attention. We take from the others what they mean for us in our life, what they have contributed to our life and our growth, no matter in which form. We take it with gratefulness. We can turn to them without pressuring them, without being in the way of what guides them on their path. Our kind feelings leave them free, and us, too. They are free from us, and we from them.

Too late

We come too late when we have missed something that will not come again. When we are late for a decisive rendezvous, we can forget about it. Too late in this sense means, something got in the way for me, it held me up because it appeared more important.

Like this, expressing gratitude often comes too late, or an acknowledgement, or love.

An insight also comes too late at times. It could have told us what would have been possible, but we had overlooked it. The regret about a missed opportunity comes too late. Above all, hope comes too late.

But the moment never comes too late. It is always there, fully there. It offers us everything, we only have to take it. However, it demands our full attention. Our full attention shows when the moment absorbs us fully, when we lose ourselves in it.

This is one side of the full moment. The other side is our alert recollection. It is outward directed but without moving. In this state we experience ourselves included in something vast and whole. We take it in and reverberate in it. Everything is contained in this vibration. It is there in perfection, in the moment.

In this sense every relationship lives from moment to moment. It reaches its fullness in the moment.

Life is never too late, and neither are the things that grow. It's us who are late sometimes, too late to take it in its fullness and rejoice in it, to be joyous now.

As for life, there is no 'too late' for love and happiness in the moment, in the moment right now.

Occupied

Occupied can mean, it is taken by someone, for instance a position. Here it means, it is taken into possession in a way that excludes others.

Conversely, we use the same expression when something is open for others and at their service, like when there is someone in an office. Occupied can also mean, please wait. For instance, when several people want to use the same service at the same time, but they can only be served one after another. A telephone connection is often occupied this way.

Sometimes a region or country is occupied by an alien power, for instance, after losing a battle. Then we speak of occupation or an occupying force. The occupiers have the upper hand for as long as the occupation lasts.

When we appear absent sometimes, we are taken into possession by something else, like by other thoughts. We are not occupied with something then, but rather by something. When we are very intensely occupied we speak of obsession. For instance, many people are obsessed with a certain idea. It takes hold of us thus that we are no longer available for anything else.

Are we also taken into possession by unknown beings or spirits? Clearly yes. Some people repeat one of their ancestor's fate, for instance. Then we say they are entangled in this ancestors' fate.

But the question is: Do the living take possession of one of their ancestors' fate, or is it this person with an unfinished fate who takes a living descendent into possession? Sometimes unknown souls are still attached to a house or a place, and they attach themselves to its inhabitants or an unsuspecting passer-by. In this way they occupy them for a while.

Some people experience a connection to a dead person who wants to take the living person into their service, like certain healers, for instance.

How do we deal with this kind of occupation? In resonance with it. This means, we tolerate their occupation with love. Together with these souls we walk in a direction that helps them to become free. This also helps us to our freedom. We become free to enter into a connection with them where we experience them as turned to us with friendly feelings. Like we supported them first on their journey, they support us now on ours.

How is it when such dead people or other beings are taking us into service for others? We remain pervious and do not attach ourselves to them. And at the same time our gaze goes beyond them to the power in whose service we are. Through this power we are connected to each other and yet also free for our very own service.

What occupies us completely? The spiritual power that brings everything into existence in its creative manner and persistently holds it all in its existence. In accord with this power we are in the service of love for many. Occupied and guided by this power's love, in accordance with its love, we willingly take along what we must and may take with us on our journey.

Where does our gaze go then, and where does our movement go? To this power, to it alone, in accord with it. Because we are all guided by it in the same way, with the same love, including those occupying us, we are all connected with each other and at the same time free and prepared for this all embracing love.

The morning

The morning shines. Something rises in it. The bright new day comes along with it.

The morning is a new rising. With this feeling we begin our day's work.

The morning is time of hope. We look forward to what it brings, and we prepare ourselves for what is awaiting us.

The morning is the time of freshness. After the night we are full of vigor, and willing to give our full effort. Therefore we say, the morning star has a golden glow. We leave the night behind and set out to action.

In a similar way we speak of the morning of life, of the time when we have just awoken from the night in our mother's womb. We are still a bit drowsy and dreamy, before we get going properly. But then we are in full swing, in motion towards the newly arriving, the full life.

There is also a morning of the spirit, as if after a dark night spirit had woken up in the brightness of reason. The Orient experienced the morning of the spirit in the Philosophy of the ancient Greeks. It is still shining brightly.

We also speak of the morning of creation, when God created the world and said: "Let there be light!'

This creation never ends. It is always fresh like morning dew, it is always beginning. We can come into resonance with this creative movement, constantly towards new horizons, carried by it, taken along. In consonance with it, we look forward to every dawning of a new day.

What is the driving force in this movement ?It is love, the sparkling, shiny love that moves to the day that's ever new, eternal morning spirit.

The night

The night is dark. What appeared important to the day is veiled by the night. Night protects it from usurpation.

We carefully grope our way though the night. One misplaces step, and we could lose our footing. We can only sense our next step.

We can also entrust ourselves to the night. Then without seeing we know the next step, we know it with confidence. Suddenly another power guides us, a power that sees.

During the day we largely rely on ourselves in what we see and how we act.

During the night we rely on something outside of us that we cannot see. But we feel it taking us by the hand.

In the protection of the night we can move differently. We are lead along secret paths, and even blindly we sense the secrets of the night that the day hides from us.

Only in the night do the stars shine, only in the night do we begin to conceive the immeasurable distances. Day's brightness is near, night's realms are unfathomably vast.

What does this mean for our life? Only in the night do we become wide open. Only in the night do we become still, in silent awe and devotion.

The day is for walking, the night is for abiding. Under the dark wings of night we find peace, we let go. The night guides us elsewhere, into a space eternal.

Where is our home? There where we can sleep, where the day remains behind us and the night opens before us.

Where do we find God? In the night as it completes the day. We find it in the night that accomplishes all, moving all differences aside. Night receives all in sameness.

Where does love dwell? She lives in the night and remains in the night, in the deep of night, in God's night.

The view

On the one hand, the view goes to something lying visually before us, a landscape for instance. There are special lookouts from where we have the best view. From these lookouts we can take in the whole landscape in all its beauty.

Only at a distance, though. It is only from afar that we can perceive it as a whole. The view is just gazing without moving anywhere. The landscape comes towards it, unveils itself, revealing its deeper beauty for us to admire. But no one may come too close, or else it draws the curtain again and moves away from us. Like when we only take photos of it.

When we gaze at the landscape from a respectful distance, in admiring awe, it may come so close to us that it flows into us and merges with us, into one.

This view is more than a visual inspection. For the latter remains superficial and flat. Sightseeing is such an inspection, for instance. We can collect many such impressions in a short time and gain an overview. But the individual pictures overlay each other easily and cancel each other out. They do not become a part of us.

The view is always wide open. This also applies to viewing our future. This is another movement we also associate with the word 'view'. Then we ask: 'What is my view of the future?' And we follow it.

We can combine both meanings of the word. We expose ourselves to the future as if it were a wide open landscape. Out of respect we keep our distance. Here, too, we wait until it comes to us of its own accord, until it opens up to us, in all its wholeness.

In this moment we become one with our future. We absorb it and it absorbs us. It has already taken us along with it, way before we undertake or even plan something.

What is our view like then? Great and wide, here and now.

Unbridled

We slow down a movement when we want to have a break or bring it to complete standstill. Unhindered, it would go on...

Which movements do we want to stop or to bring to a standstill? Those movements that make us fear they might take us into some unknown territory, too unfamiliar for us to find our way around. We are frightened it might demand more of us than what we feel capable of. So we pull the emergency brakes.

Then what happens to us? The movement stops. And with it, often our future stops as well, and our happiness, at times even our life.

What above all halts such a movement? An objection. What is such an objection based on? On something familiar. Where would the movement go if we were to let it happen unrestrained? Always towards something unknown.

The objection to a movement towards the new always refers to something old. But the new is unknown. Everything new lies outside the domain of the old.

Once the movement towards the new was blocked, it will be hard for us to get it going again. It remains stuck in the old.

How do we remain unrestrained in this movement towards the new? We entrust ourselves to it as a movement of life. It is carried and drawn by other powers that carry us in their own direction, over all crossroads, unimpeded, new every moment, unhindered. So what above all do we have to keep in check? Our faint-heartedness, our excuses, our objections.

Something else to keep in mind. With the brakes on, we age quickly. Giving life free reigns, we stay young. What remains young above all else? Unbridled love.

OH HOW I'D LOVE TO
HIDE IT IN THE DARK,
WITH SOME LOST THING,
IN SOME STRANGE SILENT
PLACE THAT WILL NOT
RESONATE WHEN YOUR
DEPTHS ARE SOUNDING
FORTH.

Coming

Everything we have, came to us, especially life. We have it because it has come. Where from? From a far and unknown distance.

Do we have our life then? Do we have it for us? Or do we just have a lend of it, for a time only? Then, does life return whence it came? Do we join it when it goes?

Our parents also came to us. We have them because they came to us. But in order to really have them, we must also take them as the gift that came to us.

Everything that came to us this way remains with us if we take it. It stays for some time, if we take it and also pass it on, if it also comes to others through us.

Every coming is a forward movement. Where it arrives, life moves on. Where it stands still, it stops. We cannot hoard what came to us this way. Stashed away, it goes stale.

Often something comes over us. An inkling for instance, an insight, or a decisive impulse. These movements inside us take us along into a movement that goes to others.

Love comes over us like this, too. Love means coming. It comes to us and it comes to others. It comes to others because it first came to us.

When we long for love, we say inside: 'Please come'. Love can only stay and be because it comes.

When love comes, everything else comes as well, including happiness.

Twisted

Something gets twisted into conflicting directions, as if someone's feet were ready to walk in one direction, whilst head and shoulders are turned in the opposite direction. So people in such disarray would be seen as twisted, with their feet they know the right direction, but their head and upper body are in denial of it.

In this way we might turn a perfectly clear thought upside down. But even in its twisted state the original thought still remains. It is still visible in the distortion.

Sometimes we say to someone: "You are twisting the words in my mouth." Something that was said clearly is turned into something else.

Why? Because the clear thought, the clear word, the clear action, question some person's intentions which would lead them astray.

A distorted attitude and distorted thoughts and words one can only stand for so long. The straight forward original catches up with the truth after some time.

People exposed to distortions only need to wait.

We also distort some uncomfortable truths at times. Afraid of its consequences we want to protect ourselves. The truth will catch up with us, too.

Distortions are a game with a predictable end. We watch them and wait for the final result. How? With love.

Annihilated

Sometimes we try to annihilate something. But do we succeed? Or does it perhaps even get stronger?

Nothing in existence can ever be eradicated. Nothing that is can be gotten rid of. Especially the people we want to get rid of, or the guilt we incurred that we want to nullify – we will never succeed in this. Nothing that is can ever not be, not even our most secret thoughts.

Still, there is a way to annihilate something. It takes the opposite approach.

Why do we want to eradicate something? Because we experience its strength, its menacing strength. Because it so strong, all our attempts of destroying it are to no avail. On the contrary, it gains all the more strength.

What follows from this? Trying to destroy it, we find our attempts come to nothing, and we become weaker. When we acknowledge it as it is, in its strength, we become stronger.

What we want to annihilate turns out to be a part of ourselves that we did not want to know about. Trying to destroy it, we are trying to destroy ourselves, but in vain.

What is the solution? Everything we want to destroy we rescue from its exile. We take it in, with everything it demands of us. Suddenly we recognize it as our own, innermost strength, as a spring from which the good and new pours forth.

Finally it makes us complete and rich. But most importantly, it makes us human.

Massacre

Originally a massacre was the action of mutual slaughtering in a battle, using all kinds of sharp poking and cutting devices, lances, spears, swords, daggers, halberds, bayonets. But it also meant the slaughtering of the inhabitants of a conquered township or city. It was always a bloody affair and a triumphant slaughtering.

Nowadays massacres are mostly carried out from a safe distance, for instance with guided missiles. In this regard it can happen without personal rage and personal engagement and personal danger. However, the extent of such a massacre usually far surpasses the original man to man combat.

Massacres that are about the lives of other people often take on more civilized forms these days, but again, still with far reaching consequences for many.

Close to the original form of massacre is the massacre covered up under the name of abortion limit.

So called hostile takeovers are similar to massacres in their effects on many people, and often they have the sense of triumph that originally went with massacre. Many other forms of fighting for supremacy also have the quality of massacres.

There is also a spiritual massacre that went beyond the extent of other forms of massacre. For instance when in earlier times believers were excommunicated from the church. Through this act they were also declared as cast out by God and damned to live in hell.

The same applied when certain sins were declared as mortal sins. Mortal sin meant, a person who committed any of them, was separated from God and deprived of salvation. They were punished with hell.

Such threats were used in many ways as pressure in political conflicts, on a small and large scale. They were basically nothing other than massacres, also connected with a feeling of triumph for the slaughterers. Spectacles of massacres were carried out in the burning of so called witches and the public executions of so called heretics.

These threats were real for all believers; all people under the dominion of the church were intimidated by them; hence the extent of the terror.

What puts an end to these massacres on all the different levels? The insight that all human beings are equal before the creative power who gave life to all of them, who loves them all with the same love, and gives them all the same right to be in the world.

What follows from this? We protect each life like our own. We support each life like our own – with love.

Free

When we feel free, we heave a sigh of relief. We can leave behind something that took a lot out of us and burdened us. Now we are released. We have before us some leisure time, time at our free disposal.

Now we can do something that has been on our mind and in our heart, to do, something we had no time for until now. We gladly give our free time to it, from our heart, with love.

Everything that can come from the heart is free. How do we attain freedom from everything? With our heart. When we follow our heartlove and meet others with this love, they feel free, too, at least for a little while.

This brings some free time, too. We relax and recharge our batteries, to continue with our work all the more joyfully.

We feel free where we sense we are welcome, received, accepted. Kind attention creates a space in which we can move freely, without fear of bumping into something. We really experience this when we come home from work and relax, knowing we are welcome.

Wherever we are exposed to extra demands we create some free space into which we can retreat, even if it is just for a coffee break.

We feel free when we experience our work as a service that is of support to others and achieves something for them that serves their life. We have the strongest sense of freedom where we achieve something together with others that brings us closer together and helps many people. This service frees us for love, and it frees us from our little self.

Calm

Calmness is recollected towards a movement. It is the calm before a movement. In this calm we collect the energies that will take us into this movement and lead us on in it. Calmly we await the right time, the recollected, full time.

Another calmness greets us at the end of a movement, when its goal has been reached. This allows us to let it be over. Because a movement is over and we let it go, we find the calm for the next movement.

The calm movements are movements of growth. They move in accord with life and love.

Calm in this sense is fulfilled happiness. Fulfilled, it looks back, and thus fulfilled, it recollects itself towards the next fulfillment that is already announcing itself, calmly so, free from hurry.

Anything that stays is calm. An old house, for instance, whatever happened and still happens in it, it rests in calmness. And a landscape is calm. Looking at it, we also become calm, knowing ourselves connected with something that abides, something in which we can rest.

The new is also calm. It knows its time is coming. Only the old gets restless when it wants to overstay its departure.

Therefore the farewell in accord with the flow of time is calm too. Therefore the grave is calm, together with the many other graves at the cemetery. Nothing may disturb their peace.

In our soul, do we also leave the dead in peace? When we leave them in peace they withdraw after some time, into their eternal repose. Whatever existed for them, and between us and them, it finds rest, finds its recollected rest, a rest that endures.

Worries and cares

Worrying about others invades them and leaves them no peace. These worries become the content of our life, even though they are about someone else. For instance about the life of a child.

What happens to us when others worry about us? We live their life instead of our own. We become a surrogate for their life.

Worries about others take us away from our own life. Through our worries we turn someone else's life into our own. We lose our life to someone else, but without the other person being able to take it.

We can care for our own life, in a way that is hinted at in the expression "taking care of", in contrast to 'worry about'. We care for our life by taking good care of it. This care is love. It enables us to care for others with love without worrying about them. Loving care makes others thrive the way that is in accord with their life. It leaves them free for their own life.

Related to the word care is the word careful. Careful means mindful. We relate to something or someone in a way that preserves how someone or something is. We take care of it with loving care, so that it is maintained as it is. For instance a precious family heirloom. We save it into the future through our care, not through our worries. We just look after it, carefully restore it and preserve it. We are just caretakers.

This is also a good way to be concerned about love. We keep it alive, through our loving care, new every day, ever new.

Spinning a web

Most finely spun is the spider's web. So fine that the victim only perceives it when it is caught up in it.

Who spins the web? The spider. She only needs to wait for a victim to get caught in the web, and there's her meal.

We also say of some people that they have the threads in their hands, unbeknown to those who are caught in them. Here, too, someone makes use of the finely spun threads, to their own advantage, in order to gain power over other others. Intrigues are such webs. We speak of woven plots.

We also weave webs of thought until an important insight gets caught in it. A yarn, a story, is also spun. When someone weaves a lot of thoughts together without arriving at any tangible meaning, we say the person is rambling, just rambling.

Where a web is spun it is meant to remain inconspicuous. Therefore it has to be finely spun. Only then will something get caught in it.

How do we avoid such a web? We move slowly and carefully. For usually, things fly into a web. Sometimes we begin to pull at such a web. We upset its positioning, to give a timely warning to someone who is about to be caught in it, to bring people to their senses.

Finely spun is the web of love between husband and wife. Both are spinning it, both are caught in it.

Our life is also finely spun. How many threads work together in it and keep it together and hold us in our place? Could we escape it? Would we escape it? Where would we fall, without these threads that hold us?

We consent to this web without precise knowledge of its design, without knowing the many threads that pull at us. One thing we know for certain: we are held by it.

We are also spinning our threads in this web, held by them and holding others. We are spinning them with love, in the service of life.

I hand over

One hands a position over to a successor. One also hands a task over to a subordinate. The subordinate takes on this responsibility, taking care of minor issues, thus freeing the superior to attend to others duties to a greater extent.

We hand ourselves over to a fate that meets us, even targets us, and in accord with it we find another path that opens for us now.

We hand ourselves over to a movement of the spirit that takes us along into a kind of action we have avoided until now because we were neither prepared nor willing to take something like this on. Taken along by this movement we hand ourselves over to whatever challenges it poses for us. We remain in its service.

In this sense we hand ourselves over to God, whatever we perceive as the reality that is hidden behind this word for us. In accord with a movement of the spirit we hand ourselves over to this reality, in everything.

Which way? We hand ourselves over actively, alert, with everything we've got. This means, we give ourselves over to it with regard to something greater, to something more. This is on contrast to a movement of passive surrender, of giving up which marks the end of a movement. We jump, figuratively speaking, on a moving train, rather than gazing after it.

We hand what is completed, over to a movement that releases us from our involvement, because this movement goes on, and we let go of all care and concern about it. Parents for instance release their children to their respective life paths and hand them over to their own full responsibility for their life.

In the end we hand our little self over to a movement shared by all human beings: All taken to the same goal without exception, there with all others, simply there.

Please

"Ask and you shall be given", it says in the bible about asking God, turning to God for something we need. We take it for granted that God hears our pleas.

"Ask and you shall be given" also applies to our human relationships, especially that between husband and wife. We often ask the other something that is important to us, for ourselves and for the other. We ask out of loving care and concern for the other. When our request comes from the depth of our heart, we are both received. Asking this way does our love good, for it is a movement of love.

When a request is met, the fulfillment is also for the one who met the request. This giving side is even more on the receiving end than the one who asked.

This asking out of loving care has God's blessing, the blessing of love for both partners.

Perhaps this is the secret behind the word in the bible: "Ask and you shall be given." It is a plea of love for many. It is a plea that is always fulfilled for it is in accord with God's love.

This word in the bible holds yet another secret. God asks us to ask of Him, to ask with love. Letting us receive from Him, He reveals to us His Love as attentive love, as awaiting love. His Love is waiting for us to be taken, and in taking it, to love like He does.

This asking and receiving is exchange, so heartfelt that we lose ourselves to Him in it, and He to us.

Receiving

Receiving is an essential movement of life. Life is happening in our receiving. We live because we receive, light, for instance, air, warmth, food, care, attention, help in many forms.

Are we always conscious in our daily life that we are essentially receiving beings?

What happens to us when we become aware of this reality?

We pause and become silent in gratitude. Our gaze goes beyond life's surface, to something infinite that we experience as kindly turned towards us at any moment. We open our soul and our spirit before this Infinite in awe and wonderment. In everything we receive and take we experience ourselves at one with this infinite, at one with its kind attention to everything that receives everything together with us. As receiving ones we are connected with everything else that is receiving, and in this receiving we become the same.

Consciously receiving we know ourselves in our fullness. This receiving goes on, for how could it end? How could this infinite ever end? How could its kindness have an end, this boundless kindness that is turned to everything? Everything has its source and its resting place in it.

Receiving we remain without a care. We live into the day as it is given to us. We take whatever it has on offer for us to receive and take.

We also receive from each human being as it is. Whatever happens in a contact with another, we see the other, and we also gaze into the beyond, to the creative power that turns to us so that we can receive from it. Whatever happens between another person and us connects us with this power, as soon as we receive it from this source, in gratitude.

We also receive what is heavy, the so called bad, also our guilt and the guilt of others, as a movement of life that ultimately serves the growth of our love.

We also receive our end as it is fated to us, whenever it comes, which ever way it comes. We are ready for what comes after it, gratefully ready.

Coming back

How do I come back? Different, changed, not the same any more. When I come back I bring something along with me: new experiences, new insights, new inner growth, another, deeper love.

When I see you again, you are not the same as before either. You are also different, you're changed. You meet me with greater riches. I have to get used to the new in you, to its challenges, to its different depth and expanse.

When I come back, we have a fresh start in many ways. We look at each other and we see that we have changed, and yet the familiarity is still there. When we parted for some time we already knew that we would both cover some distance on our path and move ahead. So we expect the new in each other and look forward to it.

Our love is alive because it moves on. I return with love.

When we meet again, surprises are expecting us. I have something to give you, and you have prepared a welcome present for me.

Who returns in this way, is coming home. Leaving had the purpose of returning.

Every essential departure ends in a return. Coming back fulfils the purpose of leaving. In returning a circle is closing.

What concerns us most deeply, we don't know. For neither do we know where we came from nor do we know where we're going to, in order to return home elsewhere. In going and coming here on earth we prepare ourselves for the essential homecoming. How? Here as well as there, equally with love.

The best

There are best things on several plains. On the physical level there one is health, amongst others. Then we say to someone: "I'm in the best of health." When we feel joyous, we might say: "I'm in the best of moods." This 'best' is written on our face and shines out of our eyes.

'The best' means here, it couldn't be better. In this sense we say of others: They are extremely well dressed, they live in the best part of town, they are extremely well of, the drive the best car, have the best job, they're extremely good looking, they're held in the highest esteem.

Who says things like that? Those who compare this 'best' to other things and admire it. They use it as a yardstick for what they want to achieve and have. Perhaps they envy others for their 'best', feeling that they are not up to it themselves for whatever reasons they contrive.

The best shows in competitions like in sports. Only one ends up as the winner. Only one is allowed to climb the top of the little staircase and put others in their place number two and three.

In team events, like soccer world championship, only one team ends up at the top. Strangely, their fans also see themselves as the best, a whole nation even regards itself as the best. Then they say: "We are world champions."

Something else can be seen here. We regard ourselves as the best ones without being best as individuals. So the group is seen as the best, not its individual members.

Especially between groups we have this competition for the best place. This competition has little to do with a special performance, but with the loyalty of the members to their group. For instance, our inner feeling tends to give our own family preference over any others. We would hardly exchange it for another. Or we believe our nation is the best, or our religion, our world view. Or our specific political system. And here, too, in our inner image and often in our outer behavior only one side can win as the best and then subject the others, as in warfare of all kinds, for instance.

The list of all the many best things could be endlessly extended. Our daily life, even life as such, is filled with these images of 'best'. Like in the field of professions, this competition goes on about which methods and goals considered 'best'.

The idea that something is best, and our desire to be or become the best, has a shining side where the glow is reserved for only one individual or a single group. But there is a downside to it, in extreme cases a murderous one. For instance when an individual or a whole nation considers itself to be chosen by God, or any substitute of such a god, like providence. This is of course, not based on any real achievement, only via divine or otherwise superior decree.

How much misery has this idea brought to these individuals, how much suffering has it caused those chosen groups and through them, so many others? How much suffering has it brought even to the followers of these superior ones, as they tried to comply with orders and rules that are hostile to life, in order of meeting the requirements for belonging to the chosen ones?

What kind of concept would be the better one and the better, even the best word, that would overcome the dark side of the word 'best'? Of course I am aware that I also enter a competition saying this. Not a personal one, though. Still, I say this word, knowing that this word is freeing for all, a reconciling and connecting word, a word of love.

This word is: good.

Good

What is good? Everything, as it is. Why? Because it is taken along into a movement that delivers it to a goal that is thought and willed by that higher power, the way it is. Therefore this 'good' is already there and also still coming.

When we look at ourselves from a little distance we sense we are in a movement that takes us further. In this movement we leave something behind that was only preliminary, perhaps even wrong, to the detriment of ourselves and others. And yet it is still a part of the movement towards something new, overcoming something old and bringing it to a new and good resolution. Without this earlier occurrence, this former mistake, the former damage, the former wrongdoing, the good of the present would not be there.

It's the whole movement that is good. We see the good when we keep our focus on the whole movement. We can only see something as bad or disastrous when we only turn to a section of this movement, in our own life or in the larger historical movements.

Seen from the whole movement which continues on, based on the past and absorbing it, everything is good, everything is in the right place, important for the whole, and good.

Why do we perceive something as bad or terrible, as something that should rather not exist?

Because we gauge it by a faulty criteria, our limited context, by the effect it has on our personal existence and our personal well being.

Seen on the whole, everything is good. Every individual fate, and all human beings. Everything received its movement from a spiritual power that moves everything the way it moves. For this power everything is good, whatever happens for the individuals concerned at any moment, whichever way it takes them into its service and challenges them.

People who were the best in any field, by any measure whatsoever, can they remain the best? The best passes the same way as the bad, victory is as transient as defeat, gain has the same fate as loss, fame and shame come and go. In the end all counts equally.

Equal how? Everyone and everything is taken along into a movement of love and brought equally to its fulfillment. How? It ends up well for all, good in every regard.

The same

It's the same, means: It does not make a difference. Where one thing is equally desirable as another, for instance when we have to choose between two different pieces of cake, we say: "It does not matter, I like them both equally." Then we have to decide which one we will choose. Even though we like both equally, we do not take both at once.

So where things are the same to us, the individual differences are still there, otherwise they would be identical. The same applies to our attitude towards differences, especially concerning people. We acknowledge them as equal, even though they are different.

Sameness connects what is different, whilst honoring the difference. It allows the different things to have their place side by side, without getting into a tussle.

Acknowledging each other's right to everyone's own place joins different people in what they have in common and what is good for all of them.

Where does this acknowledgement begin? It begins with us, when we stand next to others as basically equal. Above all, we have the same source, the same origin, and the same goal, the same end.

All sense of superiority comes to an end here, and every better or worse. It is the beginning of human love of humanity, for all as they are, wherever they are on their journey at the moment, on the road to their and to our goal.

This is also the end of the little self that separates, and the beginning of the we that embraces all.

Clear

Clear means transparent, not clouded by anything. Where something is transparent I have a clear view which allows me to perceive with precision.

What I have perceived with clarity, I can remember clearly, I can express it in clear words, so that everyone can understand it clearly.

When I communicate something with clarity, I am clearly focused on the people I am talking to so that I can see whether they follow me. This is an important aspect of clearly expressing what I have perceived, so that it also becomes clear to my listeners. So this way a clear understanding and a clear relationship can develop between us.

So far we have talked about clear external perception. Here we find few obstacles, for what stands in the way can usually be cleared up easily. This perception is well supported by the fact that it can be tested. We only need to look carefully and listen carefully. This perception becomes clearer still when we involve our other senses, too.

It's a different matter when emotions play a role in perception, for instance when a situation is perceived as threatening. Fear distorts perception, and so do secret wishes, or a strong desire, an ardent hope, and above all, rejection and love.

We say love makes blind. The same holds true for illusions, for firm beliefs and a treacherous hope. To remain level headed in such situations is difficult for many.

Here it is important to get a clear picture of the situation, to think clearly, to gain clear insights and take clear steps. With their help we overcome the limitations opposing clear actions.

This clarity is recollected clarity. It comes to us when we go towards it in recollection, when we stand before it in recollection. This clarity leads to clear action and shows in clear action. In this sense clarity is an achievement, demanding courage and strength from us, for this clarity asserts itself.

This clarity is pure. It is kindly turned to others and makes people feel good. It makes things shine; with this clarity something dawns on us.

Its light is clear and warm. It joins what still lived in the dark of night with the brightness of the morning. Gloominess evaporates in its warmth and cheerfulness

This clarity brings joy for it is love. It is pure love.

Clouded

Something bright becomes clouded so that we cannot see through it. A window for instance. The mud keeps away the brightness. It interferes with it.

Sometimes our thoughts are cloudy, and in their trail, our mood is too. A dark cloud hangs over us. This means it is infectious to others as well. We speak of a gloomy outlook, a gloomy hope, a gloomy life.

Something can only be gloomy when the light is not allowed in. Without something bright there cannot be gloom. The gloomy is perceived together with the bright. Gloom and light cannot exist alone.

Gloom is a view of things that also perceives its opposite. This view places us before the option to perceives brightly or gloomily. The gloomy is chosen by us, preferred to the bright.

Something else can be observed. The bright is active, the gloom is passive. The bright remains in motion, the gloom remains stuck. The bright moves on, the gloom hangs on. Brightness acts, gloominess hinders.

What is a good way of dealing with our darkness? We wipe it away, until the brightness shines through again. We become bright again in ourselves through this brightness, bright in our thoughts, bright in our inner pictures, bright in our eyes, and bright through our drive, our action, and our courage.

What shines brightly for us? Above all, the new. Only the old is dim and gloomy, a buried hope for instance.

How many people look at us with a bright smile! They show us their joy in seeing us. Does their brightness reach our heart? Or does a veil before our eyes dim their brightness?

One way of lifting the veil is to let our eyes shine brightly and warm for them as well. Then our gloom brightens up for ourselves and also for many others.

What becomes bright again for us? Above all, love.

Simple

Something is simple when it is done easily. It does not require special knowledge and skills, and no special effort either. Everyone does it naturally.

Simple in this sense are our basic actions of living, like breathing, eating, drinking, walking, and everything that contributes to passing on life. Everyone can do it without exercising.

Simple is the joy that goes hand in hand with this simple movements and actions of living, and simple is what brings people together. Like singing, dancing, exchanging, being there together, being there for one another, joy of living, and love.

Simple is the trust that something goes well. Simple is the openness to life, and simple is our daily happiness.

It gets harder once we want more than the simple things. Big success for instance, and everything that is more than what others have, as in competition. Of course, that is a part of life, too, but simplicity and ease often end here.

What do I want to get across with this? That we stay as close to what is simple even here. That we stay with what is necessary, and return to the simple things in life as soon as circumstances permit.

Simple are the essential thoughts that go to the heart of the matter, and simple are the words that speak these thoughts. Everything is simple here, everything that serves life and living immediately: simple instructions, simple actions with our hands, the simple switching on and off.

Wherever something is simple, we feel at ease, for instance with simple people, with their simple greatness.

Simple is everything that is pure, like pure intention, and there is something that is always simple: pure love.

BUT ANYTHING THAT
TOUCHES US,
BOTH YOU AND ME,
TAKES US TOGETHER IN A
SINGLE BOWING
THAT DRAWS FROM TWO
STRINGS
BUT ONE VOICE.

Prepared

We are prepared for the next new thing that's coming and awaiting us. Prepared, we look out for it.

Prepared, we are awake. We still wait until the time has come, for instance in front of a locked door. As soon as it opens, we press on, in joyous anticipation of what awaits us, we're all ears and eyes, and look, the curtain opens and the play begins.

We are also prepared for what expects us after the play, for instance after the play of life: death.

This time, instead of pressing forward through a gate, we wait until someone takes our hand and pulls us beyond an unknown threshold, to another land.

Here we are taken, ready or not. This preparedness is the ultimate one. Subliminally it is always there. It poses a limit to any other kind of being prepared.

Prepared for this, we are prepared for everything else, prepared whilst in transit. Instead of being swept along, we are prepared in a collected way, here as well as already there. We are here in a different freedom, already elsewhere, beyond the present. We are here in recollection. This means, we take and leave it at the same time.

This way we are prepared for love in a different way. Prepared, remaining at ease, no matter how stormy it may be, and we are differently prepared for the present happiness.

We are also differently prepared for loss. We let it pass, as something preliminary, like an inkling of our final letting go.

Thus prepared, the present takes on a different preciousness. It glows in the sunset, transient and still there.

In this different mode of being here love becomes precious and deeply pure.

Divided up

Dividing something up between us, it becomes less for the individuals, but more for both of them together. Both do something with this part and later they bring the parts back together. It becomes more than what it was before for both of them now. Spreading something out augments it.

This becomes apparent in couple relationships. And in any relationships, where people get together and divide amongst them what they have as individuals, all of them gain more in the end, together as a group or community, and also as individuals.

In this sense all of life is shared with other life. It becomes more for us and others because we divide it amongst us.

No living being can survive without dividing. We became human beings because dividing went on in our body all the time. We grew through division until the fertilized egg became an embryo and later on a human being, capable of surviving outside the womb.

As adults we stay alive because there is ceaseless renewing through division going on in us. We are kept alive through processes of division.

A mental way of turning something into shared parts is communicating. We share knowledge around, or an experience, or an insight. We let others participate in our joy and happiness, and often in our grief and loss.

Feelings we let others participate in become less on the one hand, like the pain about a loss. On the other hand something becomes more through this participation. We become more humane and more loving, richer and deeper.

One thing remains undivided: Our being – that which unites us with our source and with many others, uniting us in fulfillment.

Cheerful

Cheerful, we are at ease. Cheerful, we are looking forward: full of expectation, carefree. We take everything easy, and we are on our way.

Cheerful, we remain with the near that lies ahead of us, not giving much thought about what comes after it. Cheerful, we live for today, letting our thoughts and our eyes roam, constantly discovering something new: Joyous like children, any moment something else attracts our attention. Above all, we are cheerful when we feel like children again.

We are cheerful in nature, breathing freely, coming alive, losing ourselves in it.

Cheerful we are most deeply connected to others, like when we are on a journey together. We sing along cheerfully, we dance cheerfully, we go hiking cheerfully, cheerfully we stop off at an inn.

In a merry round we come alive, we forget many things, we become light, float above many things, we feel restored and become curious about what's next.

Joyfully we sweep others along into a joyful day, from highlight to highlight, and when the day winds down, we fall asleep, cheerfully and blissfully.

In God's presence we are also joyous, near the Dear God, before someone put the fear of Him into us, and drove us out of paradise, where He was right amongst people.

Cheerfully, we return into His paradise, like children, home again at last, happily at home.

Inclined

The inclined deviates from the straight. It turns to something, it bends down to something.

We bow down before someone who has a higher position than us, our parents for instance, and we bow down before God.

In response, they bend down from their height towards us. This way they show they are kindly inclined towards us.

We are inclined towards something when we turn to it, when we come into connection with it, when we dedicate ourselves to it, when we give something of ourselves to it, when we take something from it.

What bends this way and is inclined towards something, keeps its firm ground, for it straightens up again and returns to its full height: flexible, able to bounce back, at ease, full of staying power, like a reed after a stormy wind. Therefore what cannot bend, will easily break.

What bends, gives in to something stronger. In accord with it, it yields, and in accord with it, it straightens up again.

Thus we give way to the new, when it comes roaring along. We yield to the young that has future.

Everything that adjusts, bends. In this manner, it keeps its ground and develops further.

Love also bends. It bends towards something and it bows. In this it remains on firm ground, remaining kindly inclined and reliable.

The same goes for life as it continues on, kindly turned to many things, and still standing firm. Life remains connected to above and below. Everything in motion remains flexibly connected.

Healthy

Healthy means, something is working well, so that it thrives. In the first instance, this applies to our body. When each organ does its job well and everything works well together in our body, we feel good and fresh, awake and full of zest for life, we are in good health. Everything works according to plan, just as it should, and we don't lack anything.

We also speak of a healthy development, of healthy conditions, of healthy prospects, of healthy organizations.

Basically everything that serves life, the life of many, is healthy.

We also speak of a healthy attitude, of a healthy instinct, of healthy relationships, of healthy children, of a healthy environment, of healthy air, of healthy food, of a healthy lifestyle.

The opposite of healthy is sick. We describe all kinds of things as sickly, when they have lost their impetus and shrink rather than grow.

Again, primarily we refer to our body, and from the analysis of our bodily functions we derive descriptions of other functions and connections that should serve life, but aren't up to it any more. We speak of a weak or strong currency, of an ailing economy, of poor prospects, of a sickening environment, of an unhealthy or even insane relationship.

Because anything that is sick limits us and causes pain, it mobilizes energy to regain health. For health is our greatest good, in every regard, for health means life.

Health requires above all a spiritual attitude. Health is a spiritual process. What this attitude requires is a spiritual achievement, for our attitude above all mobilizes energies for recovering health.

What above all makes us healthy? The joy of living. This joy is active. It gets involved and looks forward. It wants more rather than less. It increases its energy and zest, it gets going, and it is determined.

This spiritual attitude is the decisive factor in regaining and maintaining our health. It sweeps others along, too, and returns them to health as well, because it sets a cycle of hope in motion.

This joy is love for life, for the full life. It is lively and keeps us alive. It connects us to our source with love and it remains in love, in healthy love- happily.

Letting be

Letting be means letting go. Letting be means leaving alone. We let something go that wants to be elsewhere, and we let something be elsewhere, we let something be other than what we want it to be. Letting be we become free of it. We don't touch it, for we might burn our fingers.

It's different when we let go of something before the appointed time, like a responsibility, a task, a gain, or a success that is still on its way. Through this kind of leaving be we cheat ourselves and others, without really letting go. For what belongs to us stays for as long as it takes to be completed.

So what do we do with it? What do we have to do with it? We complete it, until it lets go of us because it is fulfilled. For instance looking after a child, or caring for a sick person. We let go when the task is done.

It is always the right time to let go of many inner pictures of right or wrong, to let go of suspicion, to let go of our fear of losing our life, and all those futile worries.

There are also certain kinds of love we would do well letting go of: blind love, arrogant love, love that we use to submit others, or to tie others to us.

It is different with the love that lets others go and lets them be as it is in accord with their own nature. This love remains even though we let it go. It stays because it is pure.

Pure love lets go of many plans of its own. It commits to the moment, to what is really there and really possible. It lives from moment to moment, unconcerned with past or future. It is fully turned to the moment, and it does not have to wait. With this pure love we find our way to others, and they find their way to us. We find each other mutually and together, in recollection we find our way to a new 'us', we are there in letting be, there with love.

Taken

"I gave it to you." "Did you take it, though?" You said: "Yeah, yeah." But you put it aside carelessly, and with that you said to me: "No, no."

Like this we sometimes said to our parents: "Yeah, yeah." But did we take it? In the same way we say to life: "Yeah, yeah", but often we behave carelessly and thus we say to life: "No".

Once we have really taken our life as ours, we love it as it is. Only then does it reveal its hidden beauty and greatness, whatever the circumstances under which we received life, and under which we may and must live it.

Truly taking our life, we also take the love from whence it comes, the love that lets it grow and thrive, and we love our life with this same love. Only taking life thus do we have our life fully.

Is it possible to take only parts of it, just the raisins, not the dough? Only its beginnings, without its unfoldment? Can we take life without passing it on and without serving new life with our own?

Life wants more, it wants more every day. We take it in more every day, more with awareness and mindfulness, more with love. In taking it, we have it, more of it with every new day.

The full life is life taken fully. The full love is love taken fully. The full happiness is happiness taken fully.

We live taking life in, taking it fully and ceaselessly. We live it fully as we take it consciously, as we take it gratefully, happily, enjoying it to the full.

Thus taken by us, life becomes rich, abundantly rich, rich for many others, too.

And thus are we taken by others, fully, with love. We give, we take, and we receive at once, the fullness of life together with many others, together with others we have taken it happily. Together with many we take and give everything.

Late

Before we meet up with what is late, there are other things to come. Therefore we wait for the arrival of the late. What precedes it is moving towards it and finally arrives. The late waits until its time is reached.

It's a different matter when we come too late. Something did not wait for us. Late means here, we missed the train.

What is always there, it is never too late. Our life for instance, the way we have our life. But of course many things in life do come later. Youth comes after childhood, our work life comes after lengthy preparation, the child comes after conception, and old age as the last one. It is never too late, but at its appointed time.

The decisive insight comes often late, but then all the all the more deeply and clearly.

Sometimes our love comes late, and so does our gratitude, for instance towards our parents. All the more liberating then is its effect on us.

Reaching a stage of accomplishment comes late in many fields. But then it comes with increased power. For instance, the accomplishment of some enterprise that demanded all we had, or of a daring task that proves worthy of the effort in the end.

Late comes the hour of life when we have to wind down because our strength is leaving us and the world slips away. It is eventide, the night is falling, transfigured in the sunset.

Our nightfall is the beginning of the transition which brings accomplishment to what came late; the circle is closing to enter a new turn, into a different world, outside the reaches of time: eternal rising, eternal morning, beginning as end and end as beginning, as one in love.

Critical

When it gets critical for us we have to decide which way to move so we get out of the situation in one piece. Critical means threatening. We ended up in a crisis where things got tight for us, and we have to look for a way out.

In this sense there is also a crisis of spirit. Common patterns of thinking don't work any more. They don't make sense any more. We await a liberating insight that guides us out of a constriction, into a new openness.

The crisis of the spirit is always a crisis of love. Does our love remain narrow, excluding other people and other needs, or does it give them an equal place by our side and inside of us? Even though we constantly experience the consequences that narrow love has for our actions, we often lack the courage to change our thinking and to make room for this wide love. We are afraid that through a wider love, we might jeopardize our belonging to those we are close to.

It is important for us in this dilemma to submit these patterns of narrow love to practical scrutiny in our daily life. What effects do they have on our body, on our feelings? Then we compare these to the effects of a wider thinking and a wider love for others and for ourselves.

Narrow thinking is often quite obstinate. Pigheadedly it pushes into the same direction, against all obstacles. In the end it leaves a hole behind, a hole in the web of love, and dead bodies. It wants to annihilate something.

Wide open thinking invites others. With arms wide open it offers space to others, space for liberating actions, for actions of love.

In the absence of love things get critical. In the field of love there is no constriction, and emergencies ease out.

The day

The day is bright. What was covered in the darkness of night comes back into light. In contrast to the time of calm and sleep, the day is active. Things are set in motion during the day. The day is the time for work, for getting something done, for achieving something. It demands of us effort and exertion.

Some people dream into the day as if it was a part of the night. In contrast to our dreams during sleep that take us into other worlds, daydreams remain empty. They are a waste of daytime.

The day demands alert attention of us. It is focused on clear goals that translate into actions.

The day is the time of success. Success stands at the end of the day's work. Then the day bends down towards the night and calms down in it.

In contrast to the night, the day is fresh and new. Things get moving during the day. We earn our livelihood during the day. We plant, we work, and we harvest what we have to harvest for our life. Therefore we feel alive especially during the day.

Amongst the days there are special ones. Sunday for instance, the day of the Lord. On Sunday we rest, like it says in the bible, God rested on the seventh day, after his work of creation was completed. He looked back on his work and was well pleased with it. So after working days there is a day of rest.

In between we have holidays for special occasions, where we also take a rest from work. We rest by celebrating them.

Often we count the days when we are waiting for a special day to come, where something is fulfilled, like a wedding day where something new begins.

In the end our days are counted. They cede before the night without another day. At least, this is how we imagine this night to be.

Perhaps this night is the night before a new day, a completely different day, the day of rising into a life without night. We are allowed to look forward to this last day. It is the evening of all days, the end of all nights.

Over

Sometimes we say, "That's all over and done with now". It means we want to put it behind us, we don't want to look back. We ticked it off, we look into the future.

Is it really over? We are glad that we got through it, successfully. We look forward to what is next. Then what's over gives us an extra impetus for something new. What's over comes along with us as an important experience. We can build on it and continue it in some other form.

When something is over, we ask sometimes: Is this all there was? Was that worth the trouble and effort we put into it? For instance when we win in a competition. Does it have any value in real life? Was something gained through it, or perhaps rather lost?

When something can be over in a good way, it goes on in a good way. It was the preparation for the next thing that might be bigger.

This 'over' is a part of a continuous, unfolding movement of life.

Something can only really be over when it comes with us. Sometimes we hang on to something because we cannot find it in ourselves to let it be over. Something is still missing before it can really be over. The farewell is missing.

This farewell means: I agree that it is over. I have no further expectations. I no longer regret that it took the course it did, and whatever I felt guilty about, I let it be over, too. Above all, I leave resentment behind. Only then am I ready for the love that is coming.

Thus, at the end of our life our life is also allowed to be over. Our may be over, completed and fulfilled, and in deep recollection we may be ready for something new that is still a mystery.

ON WHOSE INSTRUMENT
ARE WE STRUNG?
AND WHICH FIDDLER
HOLDS US IN HIS HAND?

Consciously prepared

Consciously prepared for something coming, we are alert and recollected. We are full of expectancy and eagerly ready, for we don't know yet what awaits us. We are prepared for something unknown to us.

No one is prepared for something old. We already know it. If anything, we are prepared to leave it behind, even if only wistfully so. When we are prepared for this letting go, we become ready for new, even where we anticipate it with fear and trepidation, completely and courageously prepared.

So, being ready means, we wait until the time has come, without acting prematurely, without giving the unknown much thought, as if our thoughts had the power to shape the new, thereby doing away with surprise and newness.

Everything that comes is different to what we could imagine. So how do we relate to it?

We remain in the moment, for the moment is already here. We remain in a movement that grabs us in the moment, and we only go as far as this movement takes us. We remain empty of images and fears and expectations going beyond the moment. We remain in the moment, recollected towards what happens in it, we remain with what and how it is happening now. This means we remain empty for what comes after this moment.

Remaining in this emptiness, in recollection, we are really prepared, for anything.

Success

When do we feel successful in a special way? When the enterprise we embark on serves life in a special way. In this sense, the greatest success is a child, and later, everything that equips the child well for life, so it can eventually pass life on, too.

Wherever we succeed in something in a life supporting manner, to our and other people's benefit, this is a lasting success. In this way life is preserved and furthered.

Are we proud of these successes? In a good way, yes. Parents are proud of their children, and we are also proud if we succeed in something that brings a good harvest in some way. Here, pride is the happiness shown to others, about how we served life in a good way. These successes last because life goes on in them.

Victories are also successes; personal ones, where we were winners in a competition. Competition about the best place and the energies that are generated in this, serve life. Everyone participating in a competition, including those who did not volunteer, but were simply forced to participate in order to survive, all of them further life, even if they end up loosing and going under. All life must assert itself in order to succeed. In all realms of life we must face competition and agree to it.

Many who used to be in competition with each other, can unite, in order to achieve more in union than what would have been possible to them as individuals. Their success becomes a joint success. Their success benefits many people jointly. Then it is not so much the individual but rather the group who is proud of this success.

Many successes slip away, especially those that remain self referring, without serving life, unless we place them into the service of life as well.

These successes are personal achievements and presuppose personal commitment and hard work. Through these successes we have personally grown.

It's a different story with successes that come at the expense of others, especially if it costs them and their families their lives.

How do we remain successful in a good and personal way? When our success means that other have gained something through it, when their lives are bettered through it. Such successes make us and others happy.

Back

I come back, or I move back, I re-turn, or I re-treat. The first movement backwards moves forward. It is returning, going home for instance. Here I come back.

The other movement backwards goes away from something. It backs away from something. This movement allows us to leave something behind. It prepares and enables us to enter a forward movement. So these two are movements in opposing directions: return or retreat.

What above all do I retreat from? And where I am going then?

I withdraw from something that held me back in my love. For instance when I had wanted some recognition from people and was upset that they refused it. Withdrawing from them, I set them free, internally.

I withdraw from anything that takes me away from my path. This also applies to my wishes and dreams that go beyond my limits and remain unfulfilled.

I withdraw from my arrogance that makes me behave in ways that others take offence to. I remain on the same level with them. I also withdraw from any inferiority as is was below them. Through my guilt, for instance.

I withdraw from my own guilt, and from blaming others.

Beyond guilt and blame I remain in a love that connects all. Here I am somewhere I do not have to back away from. Here, everything is there at the same time, happily there, enduringly there, with love.

Looking on

When we are watching something, it can happen that we are swept away by a spectacle taking place in front of us. We eagerly watch a football match for instance, especially when our team is playing in it, and it is as if we are winning or loosing with our team.

Many get into such a state that they continue the game after the match. For instance in the street, with the fans of the other team, or at the pub and at home, in discussions about the match.

Where we have events without opposing parties, the audience is drawn in together, for instance when they participate in a rock concert. Often they get carried away, so much so that they sing along, dance along, even scream as if beside themselves.

People are also transported into another realm when a classical play is performed before them. They are drawn in, too; something is touched in their soul that resonates with different strings of their being and takes them into a spiritual world from which they return, enriched for their daily living and loving.

Sometimes we can see something coming that brings disaster to many, as if their fate takes its course relentlessly. We feel for them, we suffer with them, in love or fear. We would love to halt such painful fate if only we could, we experience ourselves involved in it, even though it is not ourselves. Here we lose ourselves in a fellow human way in sym-pathy, com- passion, sharing worries and grief.

Just being present, looking on, without being carried away, looking on in recollection, seeing other powers at work, and letting them be, there with those who are taken along in this movement, and yet at a distance, without intervening or even wanting to intervene, this connects us to our and their foundation. In this looking on we are most deeply with ourselves and with them.

Balanced

The balance of giving and taking is the basis of our relationships. This balance it the basis of the kind of justice that allows people to live in peace with one another.

When we balance with love, we go beyond mere justice. Loving the other person, we give more than what we received. This exchange serves our mutual love. As a response to our giving more the other gives more, too. Thus the exchange between us grows. In the service of life, love forms an alliance with justice so that life goes on and grows.

Balancing this way is more than balance that is only fair, for that kind of exchange ends with what is seen as just. Exchange with love, going beyond mere justice, binds and joins, because the exchange continues on beyond the fair part. Love is the crown of justice and takes it to another level.

Exchange with love continues also in another way. In the service of love we pass on something to those who cannot give back yet, according to an idea of fair balance. Like parents give to their children.

This exchange is serving with love. Here, love comes first. It gives without expecting the other to reciprocate in the realm of fair balance. The young will later give in the same way, passing this love on to others, the young of the next generation, who are now in the same situation as they were before, only able to receive in the beginning, and not reciprocate according to a principle of balance. But later they will balance, by serving others with love, the way they were served.

Serving is the most complete exchange. It is love in the first instance, love through passing on, love in the service of another life, in passing on life and passing on love. Here justice becomes love. It turns into the fullness of love.

More

'More' is more life. All other kinds of 'more' are transient only. The 'more' of life is the one that stays, because it keeps on going.

'Less' is less life. 'Less' diminishes life, it goes against life.

When we tune ourselves into 'more' on every level, we experience in ourselves whether we go with life. We tune into more love for instance, more achievement, more success, more joy and happiness.

Wherever we settle for 'less', we settle for less life, for less love, for less achievement, for less success, for less joy and happiness.

We sense inside of ourselves where our inner movement goes. When it goes to 'less', it goes towards our life's end and to death, to death before our fulfilled time.

What is the commensurate answer when we perceive this movement in us?

We change back towards 'more'. Only when we want more, when we start an inner expansion in all directions, do we remain in accord with life. Life gains more every moment. Then our quiet time is finished and all the empty and wasted time.

How above all does our life get more? When it serves other life more. For 'more' means more life in others and in us.

How does our life become less? When we begin to serve less and then cease doing it altogether. Then we are reduced to a slumber, we don't wake up enough to really serve and really love.

Does our life also come to an end, ending with our death? Fulfilled life continues on in the lives of those whom we served. How? With more.

Transformation

Different to growth where things proceed similarly to before, there is also transformation. In this process something new comes into existence that has very little resemblance to what was before, even though it arose out of it. Like the butterfly coming out of the caterpillar via the chrysalis. Beyond growth, transformation is an essential part of life.

We also hope for a transformation after our death. We have the image of resurrection into a creative spiritual realm that transforms us and returns us to our source. Our longing is directed to this transformation.

Do we already experience this transformation here in this life? Or at least heralds of this transformation?

In recollection we are sometimes picked up by a movement that leads us out of our body for a time, so that we are taken into a realm beyond our familiar time and space. We may experience a feeling of boundless love and a sense of oneness with it. Here, our fears fall away. They belong to the realm where transformation is still ahead of us, where we still fear our fears may overwhelm us in the final letting go.

For some time, we still return from this transformation. We move back and forth between the two realms.

Rilke describes the final transformation in his last sonnet to Orpheus like his transformation in his own death.

Silent friend of many faraways, feel
how your breath still widens space.
In the darkness of the belfry's high beams
let yourself be rung. What feeds upon you

Becomes strong in being, through such nourishment.
Move in and out of transformation.
What is your most suffering experience?
Is drinking bitter to you, become wine.

Be in this night of boundless measure
power of magic at the crossroads of your senses,
their deepest movements' meaning.

And when the earthly has forgotten you,
to the silent earth, say: I flow.
To the rushing waters speak: I am.

Our transformation awaits us inescapably. Even now, it awaits us any moment. It awaits us, pure, endlessly pure, accomplished in purity. In accord with it we live and love differently, with a different sense of ease, at the beginnings of our transformation already here and now.

Arrived

Arrived means: I have come to you. The real arriving is where other people are.

We arrive after a journey that started far way away and took a long time. Thus a child finally arrives after nine months, at its birth. Arrived where? In the arms of its parents. They awaited it for a long time. And generally in our life the most beautiful arrival is where others have been waiting for us, where others look forward to our arrival with joy.

Often it is a reunion after a long time. Then we not only arrive, but we come back and home, as if a circle is closing.

Others arrive where we are and have returned to us. They love arriving with us, returning to us, when we expect them with love.

We also arrive in a new way, at an unfamiliar location, with strangers, like at our birth. Later in life, when we newly arrive somewhere or when we come home after a long absence, we have to reorient ourselves. We have all changed in the meantime. We have to get to know each other again, until beyond the old familiarity we find our way to a new one. The same as we cannot step into the same river twice, we can never return and come home in the same way.

Our life proceeds from the first arriving to the last one. Where we will arrive thereafter, we know as little as when we are born.

Will we be expected there in the beyond? Will we be received with joy and love? Are these images appropriate there? Is it a homecoming or did we get lost?

Perhaps we never left, and when we arrive we find out we were already there, secretly.

Arriving here, we step into the same river, the river that neither comes nor goes. Here we have always arrived already, we are always there now.

Readjusted

Often we meet with a situation that is different to what we expected, to what we were prepared for. We have to reorient ourselves, we have to adjust to its requirements. This means we make ourselves fit to relate to a new situation.

Our body for instance is constantly readjusting. When we get hot, we start to sweat. When we need more air, we breathe more deeply, and our heart beats faster. When we need water, we become thirsty. When we are in danger of falling, we quickly rebalance our movements.

For the spirit it's harder to readjust. When faced with something new, it prefers to relate to inner images and feelings that are familiar, rather than responding to the new situation immediately and adjusting to it directly. Our spirit responds to more than what the immediate situation requires. It imagines how others might react to a response that bypasses the images that it has about other people's expectations. What if our spirit only responded to what is right before it, immediately changing the situation thus that it serves the moment and the present task at hand best?

So here our spirit is facing the task of readjusting the inner images. More precisely, it is about our farewell to people that our spirit is still tied up with, at least internally. They may only be present in images, without any desire of theirs to interfere at all. Often the people we are concerned about have already died a long time ago.

So what do we have to keep in mind concerning this readjustment? What matters is the moment, without the past, focused on life, on what life needs right now to fulfill what the moment offers. It is about our love for life right now, about love and life, my own and that of others, right now, only now.

Resistance

Resistance forces to think over what we want. Is it goal fitting, does it meet the requirements of the situation? Did we perhaps overlook something important? Did we ignore something important? Did we deviate from the accord with the love of the spirit?

So we aim at acknowledging the resistance, to respect it and to meet it, half way at least.

Through the resistance we find our way back to love that includes everything as it is. We surrender our resistance against what resists us.

When our resistance eases, the other resistance dwindles away, too. No one feels threatened any more.

First of all there is something we have to resist, namely the love that excludes, as it resists the love that includes everything.

Every resistance is ultimately resistance against exclusion and against the love that closes off instead of opening up. Resistance forces us to expand the boundaries of love.

This resistance ultimately turns against the claim of being better, being loved more by God, being more in God's service.

This resistance is most deeply the resistance against the exclusion from God and His love and guidance.

How do we meet with this resistance? With the love of the spirit, spirit's love for everything as it is and what it tries to bring about in the service of life.

How do we surrender our resistance in the face of this resistance, our resistance against God and against how He takes everyone and everything along into his movement of love? How do we do it? Without resistance, with the same love.

Trusted familiarity

Trusted comes from trust. I trust people that they love me, that they have my best interest at heart, that they are willing to come towards me, to be there for me when I need them.

Thus a child trust its parents, and husband and wife trust each other. They can rely upon each other.

To have a trusted relationship with another person adds another dimension to trust. I know what this person would not reveal to many others. It was entrusted to me, in confidence. This deep level of trust between people is the expression of a heartfelt connection. All the more they trust each other with love.

We can also be deeply familiar with a task. We know what has to be done in order to succeed. In the course of time we have also become familiar with life, with what life entrusts us with, so that it succeeds, and with what it does for us in any given moment, so that life remains and fulfils itself for us.

We also become familiar with the lives of others, we serve them with our life, and together with them we arrive at a shared fullness.

Together with them we become familiar with happiness, the deep happiness in a couple relationship, and with the happiness that makes others happy, in whose service this relationship is, the happiness of their children.

How do we become familiar with the challenges of life at the same time, with what it demands from us at any given moment? We become familiar with it, when we trust life in this regard, too. We trust that in all ways, life will go on, even if in different ways. Only thus do we become familiar with all of its greatness and all of its love.

How can we succeed in this love? When we trust an ultimate movement of love, being deeply familiar with it in everything we love. In accord wit it, we become familiar with everything.

Our deepest trust goes to this movement, even beyond this life and our love her. This movement is most deeply familiar, acquainted, with everything, and in accord with it, so are we.

Consonance

Consonance means, to share harmonious frequencies, resonating with one another and in one another. In consonance we are relating to each other in love. And love also means resonating with one another, tuning into one another, sounding forth to each other and together, in harmony.

We come into harmony with nature, by agreeing with it as it is, resonating with it in consonance. Thus we come into harmony with life, with all of life, and in harmony with that infinite sounding forth throughout the universe, that melody heard by all of creation, each being resonating and singing along.

Thus we also come into accord with a situation. Whatever it may be, we come into resonance with the ultimate power that sounds forth in it, too. And through it, we come into resonance with this situation. Suddenly everything that is touched in this situation, resonating in harmony with that great power, and we begin to tune into its rhythm and resonate with it, too. In resonance with this power suddenly our base vibration must sound forth differently: wider, deeper, more encompassing, greater. In this accord we grow beyond ourselves and resonate with more than what we could have dreamt of.

In this way I resonate with others, far beyond myself, into a deeper and wider love, especially with those that I share my life with. Together we sound forth beyond our human sphere into other worlds, yet still with the same base note that carries each melody: the basso continuo of infinite love.

Precise

Precise means, to the point. With this, the precise is also taken away from something that belongs there as well. Precise therefore also means, limited.

The precise is isolated, cut off from something larger. The precise is what we have appropriated in order to be of service to us, by virtue of its precision.

All essential matters are imprecise, because many different things are part of it and need to be considered as well. Therefore love is always imprecise, and so is deep insight. It makes many things possible all at once.

The same goes for perception that takes in more than some isolated thing, it is imprecise because it exposes itself to the whole. It is also directed to more than just what is present now. In what is now it also perceives its movement, that which will come of it.

All things creative are imprecise, for they are in motion. We can even say that in the precise the movement comes to a halt, for the precise is concentrated in a point that must not move, for that would be the end of precision.

People who want to know things precisely get stuck in this knowledge. It becomes less, not more.

All of life is imprecise. It goes beyond the precise because it is new in every moment.

And so it is with love. Those who form precise images of what their partner would have to be, do find an image, but not a real life person. Precisely like that they end up on their own.

Through precision we seek security, in what is well known, familiar. This is always condensed to a point, devoid of the changes that go with fullness.

Fullness is imprecise, for even the slightest progress is imprecise.

The opposite to precise is open, open for more, open for the whole, open for what counts in the end.

Open, above all, is love, new every day, meandering here and there like a broad river finally pouring into something unfathomable, dissolved into enduring fullness. How? Imprecise, for it brings everything with it.

Standstill

Standstill means, something that was moving before has come to a halt. This means: So far and no further.

The standstill is temporary only when the movement is taken up again. But things also come to a permanent standstill. Life for instance, when the heart suddenly stands still.

Something comes to a standstill when it has exhausted itself. What was vibrant and strong before has lost its strength. What used to be important does not count any more. It winds down to its end.

This applies to many prevailing trends that drew many people into their spell, many ideas that people believed in. Incredible how much many people offered and sacrificed to their ideals, only to stand before the debris in the end. Like after a lost war.

Love also comes to a standstill sometimes. Maybe it has served its purpose. Can it be renewed? Can it come to life again? Often only when it continues in a different form, composed, giving up something, and becoming purer and deeper through it. It stands still in a certain way, hardly any movement can be perceived, for it wants or expects little. But it is there, fully there, as fulfilled here and now. It remains without moving. Or so it seems. But it shines just because it is there. It shines out of its eyes.

Standstill can also mean: Arrived, fulfilled, at its destination.

Devotion is such a standstill. Stillness before the presence, just there, recollected, immovable. It has arrived.

And so it is with love when it is there, always there, completely there.

O SWEET SONG

Endless

The endless is in a never-ending movement. Thus life goes on, continues on differently, endlessly.

An insight also continues on, because it remains in motion and leads to ever new insights. Each insight comprehends a part of a movement. It leads to the next insight that carries on with this movement, and so it goes endlessly.

Sometimes we imagine the end of our earth, even do calculations as if we knew when and how her end will come, because our focus is only on one point, on our earth alone.

How could the creative source that sets everything into motion and keeps everything in motion, ever come to an end? How can we imagine it to be limited to this earth and its life span, as if the universe had its beginning and end with the earth?

So let us put an end to such thoughts, and let us take them beyond this imagined limit.

Even in our life we experience the movements of the spirit as endless, endless because they are forever new. Do they know an end, a limit? Can anyone set them a limit? When the movements of the spirit take hold of us, do we come to a dead end in them?

These movements continue on endlessly. Even for the simple reason that there cannot be a destination at which they reach their fulfillment. To us, the creative is thinkable only without destination and without end.

So how is it with love then? When it comes to a destination, is it still love then? Does it end there?

What above all else is endless for us? Pure love, enduring love.

Boundaries

Boundaries keep something out. They protect what moves within their sphere, against something that has to remain outside of them. Only within these boundaries can we really move freely, together with those who share this protected space with us.

Once we go beyond these boundaries, we lose connection to those preferring to remain within their protection. They lose the connection with us, and they might even perceive us as a traitor who went over to another side that frightens and unsettles them.

To venture out beyond these boundaries takes special courage. Standing on one's own, nobody can do it. It is only possible when beyond these boundaries other powers receive us and guide us further. We exchange one kind of connection for another.

Examples for this are defectors, including those who convert to another confession. It also applies to emigrants who were often forced to leave their ancestral homeland. They had to find a place to stay elsewhere and start all over again.

Is there a realm where all boundaries fall, a realm that takes us beyond all boundaries? Which are the first boundaries to fall there? The boundaries of knowledge and of love.

How do we get to this realm? A movement of the spirit takes us there, of that spirit who does its creative work in all things.

Beyond which boundaries does it take us first? Beyond the boundaries of good and bad, beyond the boundaries of better and worse, beyond the boundaries of our judgments, beyond the boundaries of our understanding of what we are allowed to know and love within these boundaries.

How does spirit take us across? With another love, in accord with spirit's love that wills everything as it thinks it. In spirit's other love everything has its being, the way it is, everything is creatively held in existence every moment, exactly as it is.

Thus guided by spirit, do we lose our loving connection to those who remain within these boundaries? Here, too, spirit's other love is without boundaries for our old loves.

Driven

When we are driven, some energies push us irresistibly into some directions. These energies we also call instincts, such as the survival instinct, but also hunger and thirst, and the irresistible sexual urge. These instincts redress something that is a matter of survival, they help meet a survival need, they are in the service of survival. They are creative, for they effect something essential.

The question is, where do these instincts come from? Which other power do they serve? What is so irresistibly at work in them? It is the power of life as such, a divine power. It is irresistible, the ultimate cause, the power of the source, reveal themselves in them.

We are often told we should tame our instincts. What shall we ultimately tame in them? Given that the instincts tame themselves quite naturally when we let them guide us in staying alive with their help and passing life on?

The instincts serve an order and unfold within an order. When the instinctual urges are met, life is satisfied and feels fulfilled.

Our spirit is also driven. For instance by a thirst for knowledge. This shows most beautifully in young children. They experience themselves fully alive only when they can find out a lot about life and how to go about things.

Because life is relentlessly driven on further, it pushes us beyond many boundaries that want to get in its way and halt it.

When we want to stop in front of these boundaries, when we deny ourselves the urge to live, to go further, our energies fade and with them, our whole life.

To overcome the boundaries it takes more than just our drives. The primordial power who thinks and wills our life, with all its possibilities and movements, comes to support us. All we need to do is let it lift us over these hurdles and let it take us along, in accord with it, to our ultimate accomplishment. In the end, we just drift along.

Here we are simply driven, spiritually driven, driven with love, driven by an infinite love, having found our fulfillment in it, having arrived in a an enduring creative movement, from here on carried along, calmly drifting.

Merciless

Merciless means ruthlessly disregarding people. This is how the sun burns on a hot day in a hot place, without mercy. A hurricane rages violently, human being wage war relentlessly, showing no mercy. Utmost brutality is not only unleashed upon people by nature, but also by people

Is God also merciless? This is how it looks for many people when wars are waged relentlessly, in the name of God - claiming our god is the only one – against other gods, stopping at nothing. This god is merciless towards others, like them. Woe betide those who fall into merciless hands.

Many are exploited mercilessly. Man often shows no mercy for the foundation of his livelihood, not even to his own body, let alone his spirit.

Mercy is compassion. Sometimes we temper justice with mercy, for justice can also be merciless. Mercy joins, justice, wanting justice done, wanting to be righteous, separates, especially when it is about our personal rights.

How do we return to mercy? Through humility. We feel what it would be like to be in the other person's shoes, we feel his feelings from inside, we let his heart beat inside of us.

Through mercy we become less. We get off our high horse and walk on foot again.

This way we can all experience God's grace for all human beings, and like Him, we become humane.

Special

What is special sets itself apart from other things. A special day, for instance, a special celebration, a special occasion, a special event.

Our birthday is such a special day, and our wedding day. The anniversary of someone's death is also a special day. We think of our dead on the anniversary of their death, aware that for us it will also be the special final day.

Sometimes we also speak of an especially beautiful day that we will remember for a long time to come.

What is special to us in a special way? Every human being, above all those people who are especially dear to us. We are connected in a special relationship and in a special love.

Special is what serves life in a special way, perhaps even serving many people in a special way. This includes special achievements, special insights and inventions that had far reaching effects and changed our life in a special way, like electrical light.

Each one of us has a special fate, unique to the individual, incomparable to any other.

Does this also mean that each one of us is lead to a special destination? Or are we all lead to the same goal, but in different ways? Where a circle closes, every special step towards it is the same in the end.

Therefore no one has a special life, instead, it's the same for all of all: special for a while, and the same in the end.

So in the end the dead are also the same. There are no better or worse ones, they are all equally dead. Whatever we might still want to do for them, whether we love or loathe them, in their death they are all changed, out of reach of our clutches.

So therefore even in what is so special to us we await the change that makes it the same as anything else, equally accomplished.

Impossible

The word 'impossible' is used with two different meanings. Sometimes we say to someone: "Your behavior is impossible." But the fact that he behaved this way shows that it is possible. 'Impossible' means here, not according to the rules that we subscribe to.

'Impossible' means above all the opposite of possible. We may regard something as impossible, only to find, much to our surprise, that what was impossible for us, is not our of reach for someone else. With the word 'impossible' we restrict our possibilities. More precisely, 'impossible' in an inner image that creates limitations for us.

How do we relate to this image? We cross out the 'im'- part.

What is possible we reach in recollection, and at its appointed time. Like all life, it results from a fresh movement that transcends a previous limitation. What is possible – and then even necessary – cannot be preempted. It appears in its own appointed time.

The possible is often preceded by an insight that dares to think something hitherto forbidden. A new insight asserts itself in the face of public resistance. It dares to go beyond opposition, to uncover something as impossible. Something that is essentially impossible is uncovered as it really is, and stripped down to what is really possible. This thinking is a liberating thinking.

The same goes for love. Many ideals of love go beyond love's possibilities. Only the love that is possible can be experienced as fulfilled and deep.

Here it is what is possible for us that allows us to grow beyond what was hitherto impossible, until it reaches the limits of its own possibilities. To agree to this ultimate limitation takes the possible to a good and fulfilling result, possible life and possible love.

Unlike

The word 'unlike' is often connected to the idea that something different could or should be the same. We compare it and find differences.

For instance, we speak of an unequal couple in an unequal situation. The unlikeness tempts us to assimilate it becomes more of the same.

What is unlike the familiar challenges the familiar. It shows it that there is more to life than just the same, and that the similar has to face the dissimilar. For the same is often the comfortable because it is known. What differs serves in places where much remains the same.

Unlike each other from the start are man and woman, parents and children, young and old, past and future.

Unlike each other are life and death, or so it appears. For the different thing, not another same one, is often the needed next step for the same.

The same is to a large extent an image of desire that makes us settle with what we have already achieved. In contrast, any progress is unlike the ways of the past.

Sky and earth are dissimilar. Heaven on earth attempts to make them the same, in spite of the fact that they are irreconcilably far apart from each other.

The tendency to the same attempts to flatten out what is different and it wants to do away with its seriousness and its power.

In this sense, all repetitions appear to be the same. But instead of being the same, they often reveal themselves as less. Only what is unlike the old, furthers what is like it. How can that happen? The same is taken along by what is different, to the new, and the next step.

How do we relate to the unlike? We wish for it and support it. We say farewell to the same, and become richer and more through the dissimilar.

Remaining behind

When one thing steps forward, another one stays behind. For instance, the old stays behind when the new comes.

The other way round, the old and time honored points the way at times. There's still so much ahead for the young, so the old gently takes the young along, until such time that it finds its way alone. Then only does the old stay behind. But still, it remains near for a while.

Much remains behind because it does not move any more, for it has exhausted its own power. Its time has gone.

Sometimes there is something that wants to charge ahead. We let it overtake us and remain behind, fully aware, knowingly and kindly aware, until finally we catch up with the other that exhausted itself in charging ahead. Then we take it along with love, until it has learned to move on alone in recollected strength, and we can confidently hand the lead over to it.

Remaining behind in this way we are still here for a while, here with others, without interfering, until our time ends.

Remaining behind is an essential process on life, for it makes room for the new.

A movement of the spirit never gets behind. Love never remains behind.

Repose

The calm comes before the storm. The calm also comes at night after the full day. There is a calm before and a calm after.

In repose something is being prepared. For instance, when something is being hatched. After a period of waiting it is there, fully alive.

This repose is recollected. Many things that were in motion of one kind or another, condense in it. They come together and wait. This repose is deep and wide awake. It is active repose, focused and expectant of next thing. It keeps calm and cool until action begins.

The other repose is tired. We take it along when we need rest. It seeks sleep. In this repose, next steps for something new are also prepared. When we awake from it we are ready for the next action.

We also speak of the repose of the spirit. Where does spirit derive its calmness from? It withdraws from the immediate to a higher realm, where, having eschewed the hustle and bustle, it knows itself connected to powers that are knowingly at work behind everything. There is nothing that can escape or oppose these powers. They are at one with everything, and everything is at one with them.

Connected to spirit, we, too, find composure and calm, also in oneness with everything.

In this repose the many oppositions cease. We are moved as spirit moves us. In unison with everything, we are moved in recollection.

This repose is the calmness of peace with everything as it is. This is the true repose, the essential repose. It is the repose of love.

Redeemed

Something is redeemed when it is undone, debts for instance. They are erased from the register where they were recorded. They are redeemed because they were repaid. As soon as the debts are repaid the whole matter is allowed to be over.

Some indebtedness cannot be repaid. It is not limited to a period of time. It remains in place for a life time. It is only erased with death, but sometimes even through death, or a life sentence.

Is guilt redeemed then? If it were, we would set our offenders free from our thoughts and feelings. But often we still hold their offence against them beyond their death. For such guilt to be over for us too, we would have to erase it from our own soul.

Why do we find this so difficult? If we do erase their guilt from our soul, we become like them in our soul. We are also alive for a while, and then dead, like them.

What opposes the erasing of guilt? We make an eternal affair of it, as if it could live on beyond death. To keep it alive beyond death, we invented hell, eternal hell. The thought of hell keeps guilt alive indefinitely.

I expand this thought a little further. How do the just feel in heaven when they think of hell, even in heaven? Are they dwelling in the great love? How can we experience love in our life, when sins and guilt remain unredeemed in our soul? Not only the guilt of others, but also our own?

How do we get away from our guilt? How do others get away from us with their guilt?

We renounce recording it. Neither we nor others have to repay it then, no one has to erase it. Can there be guilt before God when we don't have it?

Accomplished

Accomplished means finalized. A task is completed this way, and also life itself.

Accomplished often means more than completed. It means, having achieved its destiny. It is has become perfect through its accomplishment, it has reached its proper fulfillment.

This accomplishment goes beyond an end towards something permanent. For instance an accomplished piece of art. In this sense it is the highest accomplishment. More accomplished is not possible.

A movement is completed when it has reached its goal. Until then it is incomplete. The unfinished strives towards its completion. Therefore the unfinished remains in motion. Only at ist destination does this movement cease.

Beyond this there is enduring accomplishment. It rests in itself. Even though it has arrived, it goes on working in recollection. For instance a fulfilled life. Accomplished, it becomes pure, pure being- there.

Thus, accomplished love also becomes pure. It is simply there, there is completion.

One

The obvious oneness of everything that is and its mutual interrelatedness, appears to be opposed by the necessary self-referral. Only in standing out against everything else, securing its own sphere of existence, can everything be of service to what is other than itself.

We experience this self-referral in ourselves as our self. With our self we take ourselves seriously, necessarily important, without this really being the case, seen from the whole.

Then there is the counter movement that joins us with many other people and things in a way that we feel at one with it all. Here our movement would be moving towards the whole as one part of it amongst many others: unimportant as individual, there with everything else, together.

Through this conscious movement we willingly fit ourselves into the whole. In reality though, we have always been embedded in everything else, because everything is brought into being, and held in being anew at any moment, by the same creative power.

Therefore, for the creative source of all that is, there is no higher and lower, like higher and lower forms of life. All are in the same service, one cannot be wanted more than another. In order to be kept alive, something that came later does not need more enduring attention from this power than the most simple, inconspicuous, hidden first thing.

How do we respond to this all embracing reality with a conscious harmony? We agree to it in all its consequences for us and others. We agree to our living and dying, whether we continue as individuals or whether we are taken along and exist in this all embracing movement in a different way, together with everything else, one with everything else.

Guide to Bert Hellinger's Publications in English

Rising in Love
A Philosophy of Being
Hellinger Publications
ISBN 978-3-00-024697-5

You hold in hand a kind of prism. The light shines through it and is refracted into the far reaches of the color spectrum. The colors themselves capture our imaginations. And then there is the place in each of us that carries those colors into the world. In this way, we too are prisms, and through the varied permutations of our own understanding, these distinct and related hues can be merged into a great expansiveness. Bert Hellinger calls this book Rising in Love. What is love? It is white light into myriad variations; it is myriad variations combined into white light. In the end – and in the beginning – Rising in Love is a state of being. Insofar as one can create a textbook for this level of investigation, Rising in Love is a state of being.

Acknowledging What Is
Conversations with Bert Hellinger
Zeig, Tucker & Theisen, Inc.
ISBN 1-891944-32-0

In this probing interview, Gabriele ten Hovel brings to her conversations with Bert Hellinger a journalist's skepticism. Tough questions are met by equally tough answers – and as this extraordinary dialogue builds, the formidable power of the family constellation approach begins to unfold. Born out of the most humble therapeutic stance, that of respectful observation, this approach makes contact with the deepest levels of family engagement and disengagement.

Sit in as the logical minded journalist and the "caretaker of the soul" consider the human condition together. Here is an opportunity for Bert Hellinger to lay to rest some misunderstandings, to clarify his thinking on entanglement and resolution, to describe what he means by "movements of the soul." You may take away little gems or find that your perspective goes through a major shift – either way, these "conversations with Bert Hellinger" will energize your thinking.

Love's Hidden Symmetry
What Makes Love Work in Relationships
Carl Auer Systeme Verlag
Zeig, Tucker & Theisen, Inc.
ISBN 1-891944-00-2

Love's Hidden Symmetry is a book to be read slowly . . . and then to be read again and again.

A lively blend of narrative, storytelling, transcript material, and poetic imagery is invoked to describe, and to demonstrate, what Hellinger calls "the orders of love" and how disturbances in the orders of love create a legacy that must be reckoned with for generations to come. But these deeply embedded forces in the family system can be harnessed for healing once they are acknowledged, respected, and gently redirected.

Hellinger's basic tool for helping family members restore balance is the use of family constella-

tions. Hellinger along with coauthors Gunthard Weber and Hunter Beaumont, clarifies how this method can be refined and expanded to galvanize the energy of everyone involved toward a greater sense of well-being.

Love's Own Truths
Bonding and Balancing in
Close Relationships
Zeig, Tucker & Theisen, Inc.
ISBN 1-891944-48-7

In the three short years since the publication in English of Love's Hidden Symmetry, Bert Hellinger has traveled light years toward an even greater understanding of the intricacies of relationship and resolution. Love's Own Truths represents another important milestone in the search.

Hellinger describes Love's Own Truths as a fundamental statement of his approach. And for those who know him, clearly accomplishing this was no small task. The approach – practical, improbable, complex, and elegantly simple – cannot be easily described. It must be "seen."

Supporting Love
How Love Works in
Couple Relationships
Zeig, Tucker & Theisen, Inc.
ISBN 1-891944-49-5

„In this expertly edited book, Johannes Neuhauser brings an artist's eye to Bert Hellinger's unique approach, and shows that beneath the surface of his often-startling work there is a gentle tenderness that calls – softly and steadily – to the truths that lay resting in our hearts. It is refreshing in this era of psychotherapeutic relativism to come across the work of a therapist who takes a quiet and clear-sighted stand for the centrality of love in human life. The power of the work that has emerged from Hellinger's unwavering focus on the flow of love in relationships is remarkable: it will touch any who come into contact with it –professional and lay readers alike" Arthur Robert, MA

Editor and Co-Director, The GestaltPress

To the Heart of the Matter
Brief Therapies
Carl Auer Systeme Verlag
ISBN 3-89670-396-X

Bert Hellinger's particular brand of brief therapy can be very brief indeed. Perhaps truth needn't be long-winded, just seen.

"This book is clearly written, lucid and easy to read. Its profundity will leave a deep impression on the reader" Systema

On Life & other Paradoxes
Aphorisms and Little Stories
Zeig, Tucker & Theisen, Inc.
ISBN 1-891944-89-4

A good poem can hold the universe in a few words. This collection of Bert Hellinger's aphorisms and stories shows what happens when a healer's mind works with a poet's pen. Single truths become manifold. Small affirmations take on great power. Soothing stories carry tough messages. And sometimes reality gets turned absolutely upside down and though we may squirm in our seats, we understand something more than we did before.

Insights
Lectures and Stories
Carl Auer Systeme Verlag
ISBN 3-89670-281-5-1

In this rich collection of lectures and stories, Bert Hellinger allows us to confront without fear the deep issues of guilt and conscience and brings to light the hidden orders through which love within and between people and groups succeeds.

These stories attempt to lead us to a peaceful center – a place where we can be collected and calm, in touch with our deepest love and longing, in tune with the world, and from which our relationships can be fulfilled and our lives healed.

This is a book of wisdom: exciting, moving and profound.

No Waves without the Ocean
Experiences and Thoughts
Carl Auer Systeme Verlag
ISBN 3-89670-548-2

This volume represents the core of Bert Hellinger's thinking and insights based on his experience with family constellations work. Set out as a reference book, it gathers together, for the first time, previously unpublished material, introductions and summaries, illustrative comments and answers to questions gathered from his many seminars and workshops, as well as several interviews and one complete lecture.

The organization of chapters according to topic allows for easy access, and many, for example, "Family Constellations and Movements of the Soul," represent the most comprehensive handling of the subject to date.

Whether this book is read cover-to-cover or used as a reference book on specific topics, the authority and eloquence of Bert Hellinger's formulations and his range of experience offer rich rewards for the reader.

With God in Mind
Our thinking about God:
Where it comes from and where it leads
Hellinger Publications
ISBN 978-3-00-023534-4

The thoughts and images we create around God have their origins in hidden places. In turn, these thoughts and images have hidden effects on the souls of individuals, and deep consequences for human relationships.

In this book, the effects of these ideas on our human experiences are considered strictly within these experiences as they can be accessed and verified by evidence.

All contemplations within these pages remain human considerations – with God in Mind.

Together in the Shadow of God
Thoughts that succeed
Hellinger Publications
ISBN 978-3-00-025382-9

„This book came about without any intention. There were moments in which I had a sense that something took me into its service. In these moments I could not focus on anything else, even though other things often seemed to be urgent. Sometimes I tried to resist, attempting to get something else done, but to no avail.

Eventually I gave in, sat down, put a piece of paper in front of me, willing to write. Often I had no idea what I was supposed to write. Then suddenly a word came, and I put the pen to the paper without knowing where it would take me. I started with the first sentence. Then the next one came.

I kept on writing, and then all of a sudden the words poured out stroke by stroke and line by line. It is in this same way that I pass these texts on to you.

This is a contemplative book, a preliminary book, for the truth is forever traveling. It is love in progress." (From the Introduction)

Peace Begins in the Soul
Family Constellations in
the Service of Reconciliation
Hellinger Publications
ISBN 978-3-00-029155-5

In family constellations, the work of reconciliation begins in the individual soul and in the family. When reconciliation is achieved there, it can spread to larger groups and contexts.

In this book, Bert Hellinger inquires into the emotional prerequisites that are necessary for peace and reconciliation. He finds answers in examples from historic conflicts between peoples and cultures. But Hellinger also devotes himself to peace among religions, for example, between Christianity and Islam, as well as to peace between victors and vanquished in the Spanish Conquest, and between masters and slaves in Brazil and the United States.

Farewell

Family Constellations with
Descendants of Victims and Perpetrators
Carl Auer Systeme Verlag
ISBN 3-89670-395-1

In his years of experience in working with patients, Bert Hellinger has witnessed the consequences of the guilt of perpetrators and the fate of victims in National Socialism for subsequent generations.

This book documents the attempt to help these patients confront the victims and perpetrators in their own families and thereby lessen and even heal the patient's suffering. In so doing, all participants are allowed to speak: survivors, children, even the guilty and the dead. When these voices are recognized, they withdraw and allow the living to transcend the boundary that still separates them from death.

Rachel Weeping for Her Children
Family Constellations in Israel
Carl Auer Systeme Verlag
ISBN 3-89670-424-91

The family constellations of Bert Hellinger make visible the often startling entanglements of individuals and families in their past and present. This image allows for deep, touching movements of the soul towards resolutions previously unconsidered. Not only the participants, but also observers, are moved in new directions.

This transcribed documentation of a family constellations workshop allows readers to experience this process and join in the movements towards peace and resolution in their own souls.

The setting of this workshop in Israel, a land burdened by a grief laden past and present, adds a dimension of depth and poignancy to the healing power of love.

Touching Love, Volume 1
Bert Hellinger at Work
with Family Systems
Carl Auer Systeme Verlag
ISBN 3-89670-297-1

Bert Hellinger demonstrates the Hidden Symmetry of Love operating unseen in the lives of persons suffering with serious illness and difficult life circumstances. He guides participants step by step on a journey to discover the hidden orders that restore the flow of love and make change and effective coping actions possible in their lives.

With compassion, humor, and honest directness, he describes what he sees without making judgments, helping participants bring hidden loyalties and children's innocent love for their parents to light, guiding them as they seek to bring that love to fruition in appropriate and healthful ways.

This book is a full documentation of a 1996 demonstration workshop for professionals held in England.

Touching Love, Volume 2
A Teaching Seminar with Bert Hellinger and Hunter Beaumont
Carl Auer Systeme Verlag
ISBN 3-89670-122-3

Bert Hellinger demonstrates his masterful use of his method of family constellations to bring destructive, hidden family dynamics to light and to search for loving resolutions. His interventions are unconventional, surprising and thought-provoking. He is unwavering in his dedication to do what is possible to free entangled love, and to offer loving support when the only alternative is to accept what cannot be changed.

Truth in Motion
First edition 2010
Hellinger Publications
ISBN 978-3-00-029158-6

We look for answers to the problems in life – distinct, discrete, certain, and right. But life is moving, as a whole and in each of its parts. How then can the answers be located in the stagnant realm of assuredness? What we find there may be short-term solutions, strategies that work momentarily, but in the end, they falter, break into pieces over time or under new pressures. Truth in Motion is written in the wind; it offers glimpses into what makes way for essential insight, it invites us to step out of the narrow view and to gaze into the vastness of the all. There, right here, all-encompassing everywhere, the answers flow and shape-shift in accordance with the rhythm of life and the creative force that defines it moment to moment and for all time. When we listen beyond the details of our personal questions, we may hear the chords of enduring truths.

Journeys to the core
Experiences – Contemplations – Examples
Hellinger Publications
ISBN 978-3-00-029156-2

In Journeys to the Core, Bert Hellinger hovers at the very edge of what can be communicated. In this organically crafted exploration of the fundamental threads of human life – love, truth, God, surrender, contemplation, and so forth – he respectfully considers the understandings that lead to contracted existence and those that lead to expansiveness. His "journeys to the core" are invitations to, and reflections of, life fully engaged, holding us and being held by us.

In the course of his discussions, all and everyone are included on the infinite timeline, so that judgment and interpretation become small before what is essential. Not only does Bert Hellinger find the practical poetry to articulate his topics, he is able to clarify how his insights may be applied in everyday life.

Also available as an audio book, 2CDs

Natural Transcendence
Hellinger Publication
ISBN 978-3-00-029159-3

Defying easy categorization, Natural Transcendence is a daring book: daring to explore the essential territory of our existence, daring to ask the fundamental questions, daring to share insights as they evolve over time. Sure-footed and open, Bert Hellinger presents a confident perspective, equally comfortable in what appears to be known and in what is by definition beyond knowing. His willingness to navigate this terrain is an irresistible consequence of decades of investigation and assimilation both of the outer world and the inner sphere; in that convergence Bert Hellinger has found access to the overarching, creative force that is at work in all things. Not meant to be a final declarative statement of reason and purpose, but rather a glimpse, this book offers specific and broad imaginings of what it means for one's life to be in tune with this force.

Natural Transcendence may sit on the bedside table, picked up and read before dreaming, or perhaps in the morning before the tasks of the day take over. It is thought-provoking, and more, it is feeling-provoking; it is an invitation to new levels of profound awareness and an invitation to step into the fresh fullness of life.

Living Transcendence
Cognizing what will be
First edition 2010
Hellinger Publications
ISBN 978-3-00-029321-4

What is known is vast. What is unknown can only be glimpsed. And while many of us climb sand dunes trying to grasp some small aspect of the first, others of us attempt to negotiate the latter, usually trying to make it manageable by squeezing the unfathomable into the limitations of our understanding. The dilemma is that we are aware that there is more to life, to us, than all human-initiated study can tell, and at the same time, we sense that the mystery is unattainable, so that any attempt to unravel the riddle will inevitably prove futile.

Living Transcendence accounts for what is known and what cannot be known and even for the ephemeral nature of the thoughts communicated within it. It is both rooted and free-flowing in its impressions of what it means to live in the expansiveness of life's dynamic trajectories without retreating into the illusion of control.

Bert Hellinger has always been a traveler who keeps copious track of the images along the way. His direction is set toward the endlessly unfolding. As readers, we pick up these notes to find a radical philosophy of all-encompassing love that addresses all of our deepest sorrows and most difficult challenges. The answers are not in the details but in the complete shift from narrow to broad, from individual isolation to the assumption of connectedness.

To return to this natural state takes practice, but it first takes someone to remind us that we may have let it slip away. Bert Hellinger does that – and then he tells us what he has learned about being in accordance with rather than in opposition to this love. This state of empowered surrender is what we will come to know as living transcendence.

Success in Life, Success in Business
How they Succeed Together
First edition 2009
Hellinger Publications
ISBN 978-3-00-029152-4

This long-awaited book offers an uncommon perspective on one of the most common questions that people have: how to attain and maintain success in our work life. Familiar to many are the books comprised of techniques and tools designed for achieving this goal. And equally familiar to many is the corresponding disappointment when these techniques and tools are not effective in the long run.

At the heart of Bert Hellinger's perspective is the understanding that the problem is not in the strategies themselves but in a fundamental disconnection between how we approach life and how we approach work. The two cannot be separated.

Succinct and profound, this book bridges the gap, explaining how rejection in one area is often translated into rejection in the other.

Perhaps ...an interruption in the movement to the mother has led to recurrent self-sabotage in the workplace,

old models of masters and slaves are still influencing the current dynamics of an organization,

the entrepreneur cannot follow through because her underlying attention is with the dead,

a product or vision is out of alignment with the good of the people for whom it is meant,

judgment steeped in generational prejudices are fragmenting the work team.

More generally, perhaps current work-related quests often meet unseen resistance that is actually located in the unreconciled scenarios of the past rather than in the details of the present. The discussion here is about the deep principles of success in all spheres of life. Once this type of backdrop is in place, achieving success is no longer in the chase but in being in tune with what actually wants to happen when we are prepared.

Stories of Success in Business and Professions
First edition 2010
Hellinger Publications
ISBN 978-3-00-029328-3

The second volume in the Orders of Success series expands the discussion of how the undercurrents of family – past and current – and of historical influences affect the potential success or failure of work-related endeavors. Superficial strategies do not have a chance against these powerful subliminal forces; however, insights that are anchored in the broader context can lead to actions that ensure a depth of success with far-reaching positive effects.

Culling material from various seminars conducted by Bert Hellinger, the book illustrates the orders of success through actual cases. As business entrepreneurs, self-employed professionals, company managers, and others bring their questions to the fore, the issues behind the issues are revealed so that real solutions can be forged. In all cases, the initial understanding of the obstacles to success shows up as a mere veneer covering the essential truths.

A fresh and markedly innovative work, this is a book for anyone who seeks a richer future, fulfilled across multiple dimensions.

Topics of Business Consultancy
First edition 2010.
Hellinger Publications
ISBN 978-3-00-029320-7

This third volume in the series: Orders of Success deals with specific topics that decide over success or failure, either because their significance is not understood or because it is knowingly disregarded.

This book goes beyond the narrow frame of reference of primarily object- focused consultancy. This consultancy includes all of life. It acknowledges that enterprises and professions remain embedded into the larger process of life, serving as well as obeying them.

Like the other books in this series, preceding this one, it is also a book of wisdom. Many insights that may shock you at first, will prove themselves to be consoling. They serve another love, a wide, encompassing love. They reconcile and unite what has been separated for a long

Addresses

Online Shop
www.Hellinger-Shop.com

Homepage
www.Hellinger.com

Email:
info@hellingerschule.com

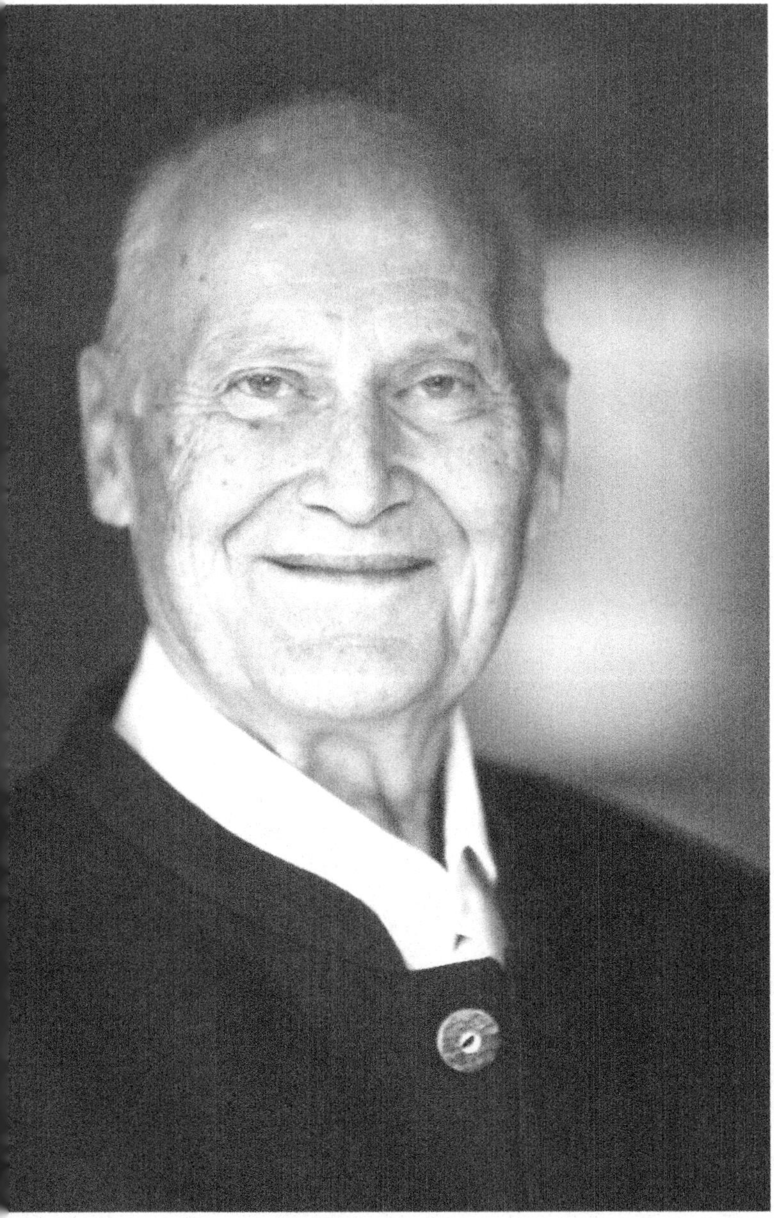

BIOGRAPHY

Bert Hellinger,

a former priest and missionary to the Zulu in South Africa for 16 years, as well as an educator, psychoanalyst, group dynamic expert and family therapist, he brings vast and diverse experience to his work. Helping professionals everywhere have embraced the new possibilities that this innovative approach offers to their work. The family constellations, which have become the hallmark of Hellinger's approach, as well as his observations about – and insights into – family entanglements and their resolution, have touched the lives of thousands throughout the world.

Bert Hellinger has written more than 70 books, many of them available in other languages, 27 languages so far, including Arabic, Mongolian and Chinese. He is a philosopher in his own right and a teacher of wisdom as his late books testify.

Printed in Dunstable, United Kingdom

91226144R00058